Heart to Heart:
How You Can Heal Your
Animal Through
All Stages of Life

HEALING YOUR ANIMAL

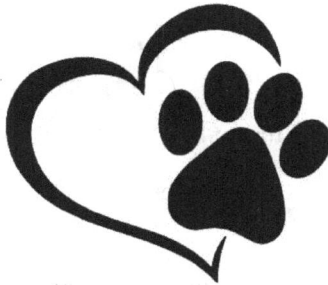

Vicki Draper

Vi Miere
Bothell, Washington

Author: Vicki Draper

Publisher: Vi Miere, Bothell, Washington

Website: HealingYourAnimal.com

Photos: by Marika Moffitt with Dirtie Dog Photography or by Vicki Draper unless otherwise stated. Animal models are Gracie the beagle and Angie the cat.

Editing and Layout:

Positively Powered Publications

Cover Design: Melody Christian of Finicky Fox Designs

Heart to Heart: How You Can Heal Your Animal Through All Stages of Life/ Vicki Draper. First edition.

ISBN 978-0-9976350-5-8

Five Important Things
Your Vet Won't Tell You

Download this free gift from: HealingYourAnimal.com/#freegift

You know the benefits of veterinarian care. What you may not realize is there is complimentary care that is optimal for the well-being of your pet.

Listening to this gift, *Five Important Things Your Vet Won't Tell You,* is going to open your awareness to 5 additional factors that impact your pet's health.

This free resource will help you be a more effective pet guardian and make a big difference in the quality of your pet's life.

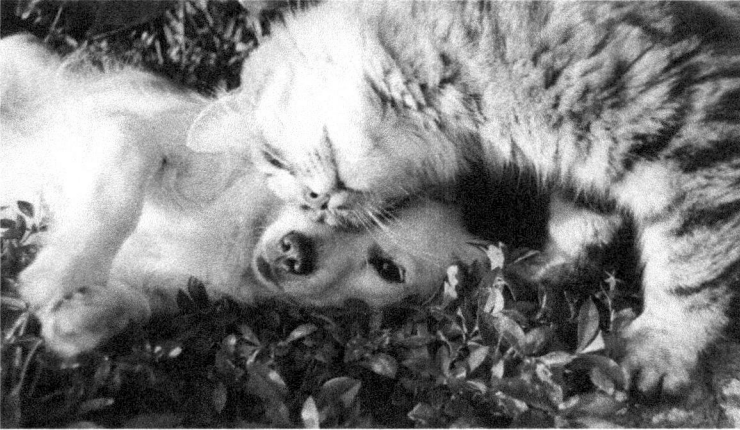

Photo from pexels.com by Snapwire

Foreword

Over the many years I have known Vicki Draper, her influence in the healing field has grown like the tendrils of a flowering vine. Her knowledge is deeply rooted in many fields including physics, mathematics, energy healing, and traditional Chinese medicine. Her hands-on skills branch out across energetic modalities, physical modalities, and the use of plant medicine. However, it is her passion around sharing her skills and information with others that has been the sunshine and water for the blossoming of her latest book.

In *Heart to Heart: How You Can Heal Your Animal Through All Stages of Life*, we learn how to cultivate the ability to consciously support our animal's health and well-being, and through intentional activities, our own.

From preparing to bring a new pet into our lives to preparing ourselves and our pets to transition to the next, all the basics of hands-on care are included here. Illustrated with stories from her practice and rich with resources, this book acts as fertile soil for the growth of our relationship with our pets.

As a practitioner and educator in the field of animal bodywork since 1986, I take great pleasure in seeing Vicki continue to redefine health for people and their pets. Vicki was one of the earliest graduates of my then-fledgling massage program at the Northwest School of Animal Massage. It has been a rare blessing to witness the evolution of both of our practices and share in the passion of educating others. I hope you enjoy the pages of this book and that they come to life in your care for your pets.

Lola Michelin, founder and director of education at the Northwest School of Animal Massage, has practiced animal bodywork for over 35 years. Her practice has served horses and exotic animals around the globe and companion animals for hundreds of pet owners. She continues to influence the field of animal bodywork through teaching, writing, and presentations.

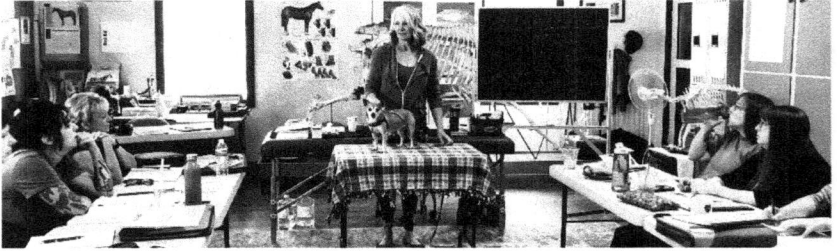

Contents

Dedication

After I fulfilled my lifelong dream of publishing my first book, there was more to say. It is with gratitude that I present to you my second book.

This book is dedicated to:

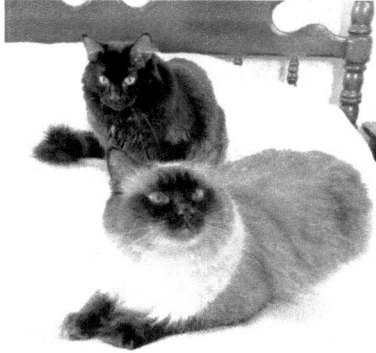

Spirit and Sapphire—photo by Vicki Draper

My cats, Spirit and Sapphire, now five years old, playful, and full of life filling my heart with joy every day.

My daughter, Miranda, for being a smart, loving person, and growing up, leaving home to go to college to pursue her dreams of helping animals.

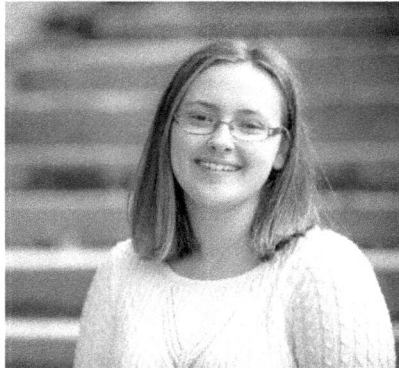

Miranda—photo by Jean-Marcus Strole Photography

All of the animals I have had the honor of being a guardian to, who have been part of my healing practice, and animals I have had a connection within my lifetime.

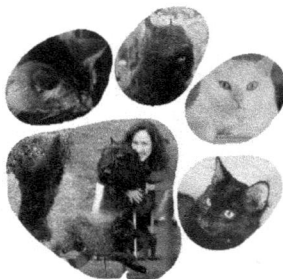

Animal Reiki Masters

To all the animal Reiki Masters who have stepped up to help make the world a better place with their light and healing.

Animals as Teachers

As humans, especially in our Western culture, we tend to be in our heads a lot.

Healing and true connection come from our hearts.

The key is to recognize when we are in our heads and to know how to reconnect and open our hearts.

For me, coming from the black and white world of computer programming, if my head was engaged, my heart was not. It was one or the other.

When I am in a healing session with animals, my heart is open and my head is in an intuitive space instead of a logical space.

Now it is a practice for me to keep my heart open when my head is also engaged. I choose to live life through my heart, and animals help me stay in my heart space.

I tried an exercise with Spirit, my cat. I was lying on my back, and he crawled up on my chest. We were connected heart to heart. I connected with him through my heart center, and he connected with me at the same time. I explored this feeling. Could I feel his heartbeat? Could I feel mine? Were they beating together physically? Were they beating together energetically?

Spirit and I connected in a high vibration of white light where time as we knew it was suspended. We melded into a connectedness of oneness and pure bliss.

It was an endearing moment, and I fully embraced it.

You can see the image of this connection on the cover of this book.

I hope this book brings many heart-to-heart connections for you and your animals, and that you allow your heart to embrace life fully.

The Life Cycle of Your Pet

I suggest reading the book and then keeping it as a reference for wellness care through all ages and stages of your pet's life.

No matter what stage of life your animal is in when you start your lives together, this book will benefit you both.

This book provides support as an addition to veterinarian care so you can do to provide good quality care for your pet.

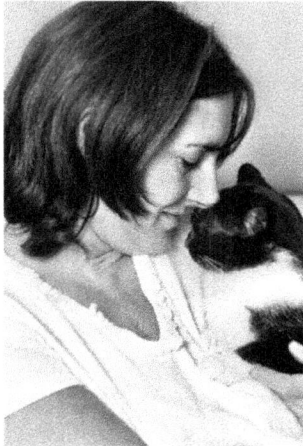

Vicki and Tasha—photo by Zachary Folk, Folk Photography

Tasha, my heart cat, was with me for over 19 years. I brought her home at seven weeks from the pound in Huntsville, Alabama, where she fit in the palm of my hand. She went from being weaned away from her mother way too early, not knowing how to receive love and pets, to being extremely affectionate and snuggly. In over 19 years, we had a lot of life together, moving across country to the Seattle Area, to the Bay Area, where she loved the warmer weather, and back to the Seattle Area. Our life included my marriage, pregnancy, the birth of my daughter Miranda, my change of career, and divorce.

When Tasha was diagnosed with kidney disease at 13, my heart sank. Then I applied natural healing techniques that kept her living with a good quality of life for six more years. From time to time she would start suffering and need extra boosting support with the healing techniques for her body to rebound back to thriving. I did not have to give her the IV drips of fluids that many cats with kidney disease require. I am convinced she lived to over 19 and with a better quality of life because of these techniques.

Then, when it was her time to die, I was with her at the veterinarian's office until the end. I took her in on her favorite blanket. I had tears in my eyes, sharing love with her to her last breath. It was hard to say goodbye. The veterinarian was waiting for me to give the go-ahead to put her to sleep. When I let out a deep breath and said, "Okay, I am ready," Tasha took her last breath. She died before the sedative or euthanasia shots were given. We were in sync with her death. I was grateful for every moment with her.

I'd like to help you have more quality of life with your precious pet with the techniques you will learn in this book, which builds on the foundations discussed in my first book *Bridging True Love Connection & Healing Between You and Your Animal.*

If you are reading this book, *Heart to Heart: How You Can Heal Your Animal Through All Stages of Life* as the first book in the series, the techniques can be learned here and deepened when reading *Bridging True Love Connection & Healing Between You and Your Animal* next.

Definitions

Acupoint

Acupressure points that lie along meridians, or channels, in your body and your animal's body.

Acupressure

As a certified animal acupressurist for large and small animals (and people), I incorporate some acupressure points for you and your animal's highest healing benefit.

With acupressure, you only need a light touch. Actually, the weight of a nickel is all you have to use to make a difference and engage the acupressure points.

I invite you to get a nickel and place it on your fingertip to feel the weight. I then invite you to place the nickel on the back of your hand to experience how it feels. Next, place it in the palm of your hand and feel the weight of it. This will help you gauge your pressure when using the acupressure techniques.

Acupressure techniques use the tips of your fingers to engage each point. Some people use the thumb, and some use the index finger. I like to use the middle finger. It adds extra compassion energetically to the session.

When you apply pressure, begin slowly and lightly. When the muscle or the animal begins to resist or become tense, stop the pressure, relax a little, and hold the point for five seconds.

Acute

An acute injury is a sudden, sharp, traumatic injury that causes pain.

Chronic

Pain (an unpleasant sense of discomfort) that persists or progresses over a long period of time.

Cun

Units of measure in Traditional Chinese Medicine

(TCM). A cun is a proportional unit of measurement that takes the individual proportions of each body into consideration. To measure your pet's cun, three cun is the distance between (the width of) the scapula between the cranial and caudal border. Divide that by three for one cun.

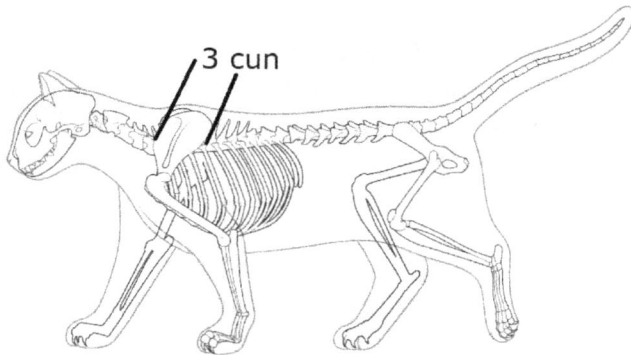

3 cun

Effleurage

A French word meaning "to skim" or "to touch lightly on" is a massage stroke used in Swedish massage to warm up the muscle before deep tissue work. This is a soothing, stroking movement used at the beginning and the end of the massage. The weight of pressure for effleurage is the weight of one pound of pressure, moving the skin in a slow, steady gliding fashion.

Essences

A substance considered to possess a high degree of the predominant qualities of a natural product (as a plant or drug) from which it is extracted (as by distillation or infusion).

"Healing Your Animal and Healing You" (formerly called Vi Miere) essences are created and handcrafted using the healing properties of crystals, minerals, flowers, and nature.

Friction

A massage technique that targets deep tissue. It is used to increase circulation and release areas that are tight. The weight of pressure for friction is one to two pounds of pressure, working back and forth to create heat and flexibility.

Gliding

A linear friction stroke following the line of the muscle, which is used to increase circulation and release tight muscles. The weight of pressure for gliding is one to two pounds of pressure, following fibers of muscle to lengthen fibers.

Healing Your Animal Session

You and your animal are together with the intent for a healing session using the techniques from this book.

Massage

Massage therapy is a type of treatment in which a trained and certified medical professional manipulates the soft tissues of the body—muscle, connective tissue, tendons, ligaments, and skin—using varying degrees of pressure and movement. It can be effective for reducing the symptoms of disorders or pain in the muscles and nervous system, and it is often used to reduce stress. Massage is generally considered part of complementary and integrative medicine.

Master Points

Master Points are acupressure points that powerfully affect a specific region.

Meridians

Invisible energy pathways or channels that run through the body. Our vital life energy or "chi" is thought to flow along these meridians. Anything that disrupts the smooth flow of chi, making the body out of balance, is said to cause illness.

Passive Touch

As a licensed animal massage practitioner for large and small animals (and people), I incorporate the passive touch massage stroke for your and your animal's highest healing benefit.

With the passive touch massage stroke you will be learning, you will only need a light touch. A gentle touch while engaging your animal's body will stimulate the circulatory system, muscles, and tissues for optimal health.

You are invited to participate by sharing your experiences on the Healing Your Animal Facebook group as you read and do the techniques in this book.

Petrissage

To knead, lift, and squeeze tissue from underlying structures. Kneading involves the manipulation of tissue with the fingers and thumb; motion can be in any direction. The pressing of muscle fiber, either between the fingers and thumb or against the underlying skeletal surfaces, releases the waste products stored in the tissue, which allows the inflow of fresh, oxygenated blood. This warms the tissue, helping the muscle to relax and perform more efficiently. This stroke can have heavier pressure; three pounds on loose skin areas such as the neck, and lighter pressure (one pound) on shallow regions such as the back and ribs.

Pressure

To understand what one and two pounds of pressure feels like for you, hold something that weighs one pound, get a feel, then hold something that weighs two pounds and see how that feels. Another method to help determine the weight of one and two pounds of pressure is to use a digital scale and learn to apply pounds of pressure based on the results.

Raking

A cross-fiber massage stroke (crossing the fibers of the muscle) where cupped fingers are dragged across the ribs. The weight of pressure for raking is one pound of pressure.

Reiki

A form of alternative medicine called energy healing. "Reiki practitioners use a technique called palm healing or hands-on healing through which universal energy is said to be transferred through the palms of the practitioner to the patient in order to encourage emotional or physical healing" (Wikipedia definition). Dr. Oz, on his national television show January 6, 2010, stated that Reiki was the number one alternative healing medicine for people. Reiki works the same way with animals. To perform Reiki, you receive a Reiki attunement from a Reiki Master.

Sifting

A muscle or muscle fiber is grasped between the fingers and thumb, which are then drawn cross-fiber to the muscle's edge. This technique is used mostly on the upper legs. The weight of pressure for sifting is one to two pounds of resistant pressure between the fingers when lifting the skin.

TCM

Traditional Chinese Medicine

Ting points

Acupoints that are at the beginning or ending of the major meridians. There is one ting point for each meridian. They are located on dogs' and cats' front and hind legs.

Vi Miere

Healing Your Animal's original company name when the Vi Miere essences were created for healing support with people and animals. My daughter, Miranda, was two years old at the time. It is a fancy letter combination of our two names, representing the courage to always follow your heart, happiness, and dreams no matter what.

CHAPTER 1

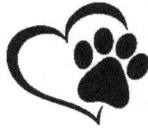

Preparing for Life with a New Pet

WHETHER THIS IS THE FIRST time you have considered adopting a pet or you have had pets before, this information may be beneficial to you.

We will start with the following questions:

- How do I decide when to get a pet?

- Which pet is the best fit for me, my family, and my lifestyle?

When you bring your new animal home, you want to take the best care of your animal. You pick out nutritious food, provide warm shelter, clean water, safe toys, and get a veterinarian wellness check-up, now what?

My intent for this section is to address another layer, going beyond the basics of what to consider when adding a new pet to your family.

Adding a new pet member is a big deal. You are taking a new pet into your home, committing to being responsible for their well-being for their entire life. I call you their animal or pet guardian.

You are making sure your pet is honored in how he or she is most comfortable with your family, your friends, and your community.

For the purposes of this book, we are discussing cats and dogs.

First appearances are not always correct, even with animals. You must consider the environment.

When Miranda and I adopted our cats Spirit and Sapphire, they were four months old. We walked into MEOW Cat Rescue & Adoption Center, where we saw Sapphire. Our first impression was she was a beautiful seal point Siamese kitten with blue eyes (that's why we named her Sapphire). Miranda and I said she was for us; she was beautiful and playful.

Kittens younger than six months old need to be adopted in pairs for socialization. To bring Sapphire home meant we had to get another kitten.

Sapphire had three littermates for us to pick from.

Miranda and I sat with the four kittens from the litter in a playroom. Spirit was hiding in the corner behind a chair while the other three were out playing with us.

My first impression was that he was not for us.

As Miranda and I sat playing with the three kittens that were active, engaging, and playful, Spirit came out from under the chair, walked into my lap, and nudged against me. He then made his way for Miranda to nudge against her. He was the only kitten to engage and connect with us like that. I knew then he was the one for us.

If we had rushed our decision, we would have missed out on this beautiful, loving, connecting addition into our family and lives.

After we got him home, outside of the shelter environment, he was remarkably loving and much more confident.

Using the techniques I teach with Spirit and Sapphire's adoption process made a big difference.

After Miranda and I had played with Spirit and Sapphire at the shelter and knew we were adopting them, we went home to cat-proof our house before bringing them home.

I started communicating with them while they were still at the shelter. I let them know they were coming home with us, and when that would be.

❧ Your Essence Experience ❧

*For extra support with Spirit and Sapphire, I sprayed the Healing Your Animal **Serene** and **Protection** essences into the empty crate before picking them up to provide calming and feeling safe. The essences are a natural, simple, effective, easy-to-use way to calm and feel safe. Simply spray the essence three times in the air around your animal or their crate to receive calming support.*

Using the essences also calmed Miranda and me down on the ride to pick up Spirit and Sapphire, as we were overly excited. And during the car ride home the kittens were so relaxed that they fell asleep. They were also so comfortable in our home that we got plenty of sleep our first night with them and every night following. It was like they had always been a part of our household.

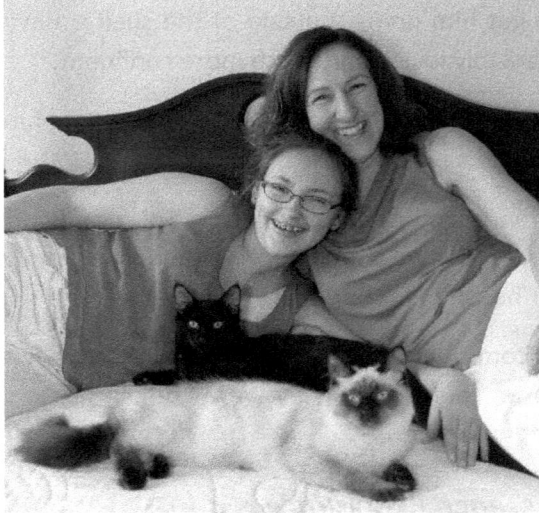

Miranda, Vicki, Sprit, and Sapphire—photo by Jill Labberton, Jill Labberton Lifestyle Portraits

Spirit and Sapphire are six months old in this picture, symbolizing the balance and peace of their new lives.

Temperament

It is important for you to get clear on what it is you are looking for in a cat and in a dog.

- Do you need hypoallergenic?

- Do you want a cuddler, a lap warmer?

- Do you want a pet that is easy to care for?

- Do you want a pet that is social?

- For a dog, do you want a running buddy?

These answers will affect your pet choice.

A border collie is a high-energy, high-maintenance breed of dog who needs active exercise every day. A Bichon Frise is a lower-energy dog that is happy with short walks and will snuggle in your lap.

Are you picking out a cat or dog because they look cute? Be careful you understand the cat or dog's personality before you take them home. You cannot change their personality. Just because they are cute does not mean you will be happy with them once you get them home. It is much more important to identify the family's needs and expectations rather than base your decision on what the animal looks like.

There are many breeds to review to see what fits your lifestyle.

Pet Care

Who will do the daily care for your pet? If you are thinking your children will, it is important to be realistic and know you need to be the ultimate responsible person overseeing your pets' care.

Purebred or Mutt?

For dogs, decide if you want a purebred dog, a designer dog, or a mutt. Then you can decide where to get your dog, from a breeder or from a shelter or a rescue organization.

Technically, a **purebred cat** is one whose ancestry contains only individuals of the same breed. A pedigreed **cat** is one whose ancestry is recorded but may have ancestors of different breeds.

A purebred dog typically refers to a dog of a modern dog **breed** with a documented pedigree in a studbook and may be registered with a **breed** club that is possibly part of a national kennel club.

Where to Adopt

If you want a purebred cat or dog, and you desire to support rescuing a cat or dog, there are pure-breed rescue organizations. Sometimes this is especially important if you want to minimize allergies as some cats and dogs are more hypoallergenic than others.

Many purebred dog rescue organizations are run out of homes and foster care. These provide environments more settling for the dogs. I did a lot of work with the Boston Terrier Rescue Group in Seattle. It was rewarding to provide care, see the calming effects, and help the dogs get a good start in their new life.

Rescue

When you are choosing to rescue a cat or dog, you can find many good shelters that care about the lives of the animals and desire for them to have a good home. Most of the time, you find mixed-breed cats and dogs at shelters.

Shelters do what they can to take good care of the animals. By nature, most shelters are very stressful environments for the animals. Animals are in cages, not knowing what is going on, all in the same room as other animals, scared and afraid. No matter how good the care is, cages are not a relaxing place for them. Know that a cat's or dog's temperament in a shelter can be different once they are in your home. A frightened cat or dog can become more relaxed and confident in the right setting. I am grateful for the people who share their love and take good care of animals in this phase of their lives.

Early on in my career, I volunteered at the Seattle Humane Society to give back and gain experience with various temperaments and breeds. They had me work with dogs that were having trouble being adopted. I gave them massage and loving attention, and the next week when I showed up, those pets were adopted. That was rewarding.

Julia Szabo featured my work with the Seattle Humane Society in her book, *The Underdog: A Celebration of Mutts*. Julia's book celebrates the unbreed, the one-of-a-kind mutt.

I have also supported and worked with the cats of the Feral Care Sanctuary in Bothell, WA. My Reiki II students get to support cats in the sanctuary with Reiki healing as they are learning how to do distance healing. In addition, my Reiki Master students get a field trip to the sanctuary to learn and support the cats at the Master Reiki level.

According to Nancy Howard, founder and director of Feral Care,

"Our sanctuary is designed for cats that do not have other choices. Their habitat is being destroyed, they have come to rely on people feeding, or the person that has been feeding has passed away or moved. We often end up with cats from animal control or veterinarians that have been brought in injured and you do not know where their habitat is. We get cats into our sanctuary that different rescues cannot socialize to a point where they are truly adoptable. We have social cats that come to us as well. For instance, they are cats that are chronic house soilers or hair-trigger aggression, cats that are much more difficult, we call these cats "unadoptable."

We put these cats through their paces in our store Whole Cat and Kaboodle to see if we can correct the situation so they can be adoptable.

We have a really good success rate of adoptions."

I have heard people say they do not want a rescue animal because they have issues.

Generally, rescue animals have a rough start in life, some more than others do. It is hard for them to feel safe and confident in their surroundings, not knowing when they will be moved again or worse, beaten or abused. It is important to understand their viewpoint so you can give them a good start in their new home with you.

The extra layers of issues with rescue animals are easily managed when you know how to help them. My intention in this book is to empower you with some techniques to get you started on a good healthy path with your four-legged family members.

The techniques in my first book, *Bridging True Love Connection & Healing Between You and Your Animal* are another great resource, where the techniques focus on supporting behavioral issues.

Puppy Mills

When you acquire your cat or dog through a pet store or from an online source such as Craigslist, you may be supporting kitten and puppy mills. And you may be getting a pet with bigger health risks.

If you are restricted from having an in-depth interview for your new pet before being allowed to adopt it, it may be a backyard breeder, and most likely, you are dealing with a kitten or puppy mill. Be mindful when you look through kitten and puppy ads. I personally responded to an ad once where I inquired about a golden retriever puppy by leaving a voice message. I received a voicemail a little while later saying my puppy was ready. That was the only interaction we had. Wow, not a conscientious puppy breeder. I did not return their call.

I did get a golden retriever from a backyard breeder, before I learned about good breeders. Sophie was her name. I brought her home at eight weeks old. I would take her on walks, and she would sit down and would not budge. At first, I thought it was behavioral. I took her to the veterinarian to get checked out, and it turns out she had a serious heart problem. She only lived a few months after that. Such a heartache, bonding with her and having all her puppy love around, and then she was gone. Even though we had a short time together, Sophie gave me a priceless memory. During her time with me, I was pregnant with Miranda. I fell down the stairs and jammed my finger as I was protecting Miranda from the fall. I was so worried I had hurt my baby. I was sobbing. Sophie, with her big brown eyes and puppy joy and excitement, was so happy to see me. Receiving her puppy love surrounded me with unconditional love. It was so precious. I am so grateful to her for sharing this lesson with me.

Breeders

Not all breeders are created equal. If adopting from a shelter is not for you, and you really want a purebred cat or dog, it is important to find a reputable breeder.

Good breeders take good care of the mother during pregnancy, and the kittens and puppies when they are born. Good breeders are breeding for the integrity of the bloodline being preserved, not for making money.

A good breeder health tests their queen cat or bitch dog, as does the tomcat or stud dog guardian, so they can minimize passing on known unhealthy traits.

Good breeders are in it for the long haul. Your kitten or puppy generally comes with a guarantee. If your kitten or puppy needs to be rehomed for an unforeseen circumstance, the breeder will take back your kitten or puppy and make sure he or she gets to a new good home.

The reason some purebred cats and dogs are priced the way they are is because of the cost of good care. There are also breeding costs that are variable. There can be semen collection, artificial insemination, travel, etc. If there are complications, veterinarian costs go way up.

Other costs that go into producing healthy animals include wellness veterinarian trips, temperament testing, providing good quality food, and healthy socialization. Breeders also spend time interviewing potential animal guardians to make sure they have the right environment for the breed of kitten or puppy.

Purebred dogs can have issues too, depending on socialization and conditions of early upbringing in the first eight to twelve weeks of life.

I have had multiple clients who received purebred dogs that were not properly socialized, and it is a journey to help them not be so skittish and acclimate into your life.

"I cannot thank Vicki enough for all her help and guidance with my beautiful Ozzie. Poor guy was so antisocial and timid when we first brought him into our home. She was able to really connect with him and reassure him that he was so very loved and wanted by us. Vicki just kept reaffirming to him that he was in his "forever" home. I know we still have some time for Ozzie to completely come out of his shell, but the trust in us and the confidence he is showing us has just been amazing. Thank you so very much for opening his world up, Vicki."

—JoAnne McCormick Seattle, WA

Selecting Your New Pet Member with Your Existing Pets in Mind

Now that you have narrowed down the type of pet, temperament, and lifestyle, it is time for the actual selection of your new pet.

For behavioral and health issues that animals may have when they are first adopted, be sure to check out the Adoptions/Rescues section in Chapter 5.

To help ease stress when selecting a new pet family member:

Introducing a New Cat to Your Other Cat(s)

If you have existing cat(s), get their opinion from an animal communicator before bringing another animal into your home. This can save you a lot of stress before getting your new animal companion.

It is very common when you have two animals in the household and one pet passes that you think the other pet is lonely. This is not always the case.

It is important to ask yourself if it is really you who wants a new cat/kitten.

I was once called in for a client concerning her cat, Stitch. It had been two years since her companion, a cat named Leloo, had passed. Stitch did not respond well to his guardian bringing home Domino, another cat. The family had tried and tried to make it work with Stitch and Domino, and ended up having to find Domino another home. They felt a lot of sadness and heartache. It had been a while, and the guardian decided to try again. Her friend was fostering two kittens, so she wanted to see how Stitch related and responded to kittens. That also did not go well.

This is when she contacted me, wanting to know what was going on with Stitch. She really wanted to bring another cat into the family. Stitch was being clingy, and she wanted to understand him.

It turns out that Stitch was trying to help his guardian work out some things about Leloo's passing before he was ready to have another cat live with them. He was trying to tell her. She was getting annoyed because Stitch was coming up to her face a lot, and she did not understand. She was thinking Stitch was being very needy, but he was really trying to connect with her to help her (and to get some attention and bond at the same time). It turns out the guardian was still harboring grief from Leloo's passing. That came out in our session. Stitch was heard; he was taking care of his guardian. She was able to release the pent-up grief and understand that Stitch was helping her.

Then Stitch was ready to discuss bringing another cat into the household. His request was he wanted to choose so it would be the right temperament for him (and that is fair, it is his family too).

Communicating with Stitch, we determined it would need to be an older cat, not a kitten, so they could have compatible energies.

It is important to listen to your pet and work together so you can both have what you want.

Include your pet in the selection of the new pet process. Let them help pick your new four-legged family member. This way, it will save you lots of heartache, lots of stress, and everyone can be happier.

Stitch and his guardian are now on the same page of the journey for getting a new cat family member.

Introducing a New Dog to Your Other Dog(s)

If you have an existing dog in your family, take them with you to help with the decision in selecting your new dog.

You need to pause and ask yourself, is it **you** really wanting the puppy? You might think it is for your existing pet, such as an older dog needing a puppy to help him play.

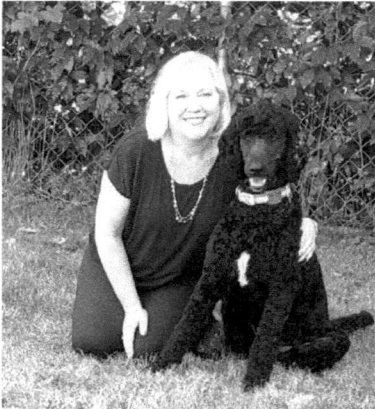

Heidi and Rocky—photo submitted by Heidi Jellerson

When Heidi adopted one-year-old labradoodle Rocky, Heidi was thinking Rocky would want a playmate, and that she needed to get another dog. When I asked Rocky about it, Rocky was clear he wanted to be the only dog in the household. Heidi listened.

When her friend had an emergency, Heidi took in Fergus (a small terrier dog) for a couple of nights (who Rocky knows and has played with multiple times). Rocky started acting out. He was getting into the trash when he normally did not. He started chewing shoes again and renewed his vigor by barking at squirrels and bunnies. Because of Fergus' insecurities and wanting to be close to Heidi, Rocky was not getting the same level of attention he was used to.

We had our regular session occur on Fergus' last day of staying with them. Checking in with Rocky, he was out of sorts. As soon as I told him it was temporary, he settled. Heidi knows for sure Rocky is happy being the only dog in the household. In addition, she knows if she needs to have another dog in the house, it will be highly beneficial to have a communication session with Rocky to smooth the stay for everyone.

Adding Additional Animals to Your Home

Your animals have feelings and know what they like and do not like. It is important to honor that fact and their opinions and preferences.

Since I have only cats at home, I am always borrowing dogs for demonstrations in my business to help educate people. Recently, I thought it would be good for me to get my own dog to help me as a demo dog. In checking in with my cats, Spirit and Sapphire, they said an emphatic "NO!" Therefore, I will honor their wishes, as I choose to keep them happy and have harmony in my household over my desire to add a dog and the stress it would cause in our household.

In the future, if I do have a dog, that means Spirit and Sapphire changed their minds and were on board with the decision.

It is common for people who have an older cat or dog to think they need a kitten or puppy for the older cat or dog to play with. Most of the time, that is the last thing your older cat or dog wants or needs.

I learned this the hard way. When Tasha was still alive at age fifteen, a seven-week-old feral kitten came to my doorstep meowing loudly. I felt called to rescue him. I trapped him with a live squirrel trap that a friend loaned me, named him Beau, domesticated him, and took him in to live with us. Tasha tolerated Beau, but Beau was too boisterous and antagonized Tasha. It was not fun realizing these were Tasha's older years, and she was not having quality years with Beau around.

When I adopt a pet, they are with me for life. Miranda, my daughter, developed allergies to animals, and she was having major asthma attacks, ending up in emergency rooms from living with two cats. I found myself, for the first time in my life, having to rehome a pet. I found Beau a good home, so I knew he was truly okay. Miranda was able to have a healthier environment for her needs, and Tasha got to live out her years more settled and comfortable being the only cat. This was the best outcome I could have hoped for in this situation.

Integrating Pets

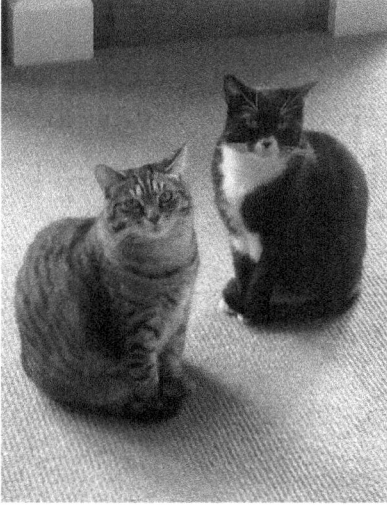

Vincent and Pablo—photo submitted by Sally McKenzie

"I was dealing with constant stress because our two cats, Vincent and Pablo, weren't getting along. Pablo was very dominant and aggressive, and Vincent, who is very shy, would spend the entire day hiding, living in constant isolation and fear. Since I have been working with Vicki, the whole mood of our household has changed. Vincent is much more confident than he used to be, and it is clear that he is more at ease and happy in the house. Pablo is now less of a bully and is starting to use more of his energy for playing and enjoying life verse negative behavior. I even see the two cats sleeping together and grooming each other occasionally. I feel much more relaxed and productive during the day, as I'm not constantly worried about the boys, and I'm confident leaving them alone together when I have to travel."

—Sally McKenzie, Seattle, WA

With Spirit and Sapphire, I learned that kittens adopted in pairs before they are six months old is best for their development and socialization. Unfortunately, not all shelters require this.

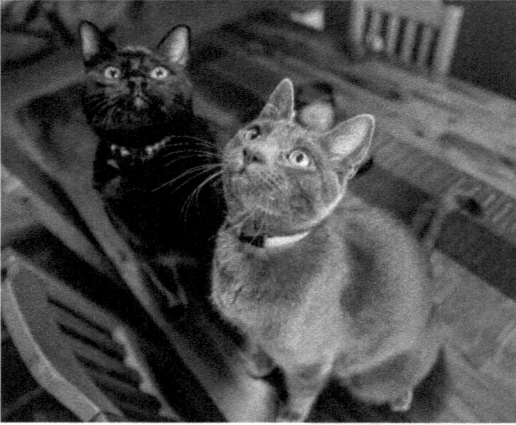

Sascha (gray) at 7 months old and Eliot (black) at 11 months old—photo submitted by Michael Poggenburg

Michael adopted an eight-week-old kitten he named Sascha.

Sascha was extremely active and wanted a constant playmate. Michael, as conscientious cat guardian, was unsettled by how much attention Sascha needed. He reached out to me to get information to help Sascha and understand her better.

When I shared that young kittens are better socialized when adopted in pairs, he adopted another six-month-old kitten, Eliot, when Sascha was eleven weeks old. This made Sascha happy. Michael was not able to find any information on how to integrate an older kitten with a younger one, so he was grateful I could help him with this part too.

The first day was an adjustment. They did hiss and paw at each other and then played together as they established how to be new house- and playmates. Eliot had come from an environment where there were only older cats, and now he was living in a new place with a younger kitten to get used to.

After a few days, the kittens were cuddling. And after two weeks, the two kittens were rumbling and tumbling, playing together, and

Michael could get some work done and get better sleep. Due to the age and temperament of the kittens, they integrated quickly.

Even when it is a good decision to add a new pet with an existing pet in your household, know that sometimes it takes more work to integrate pets. There is an adjustment period when you introduce a new pet. If you have another pet already, it is best to introduce them slowly. Give them space away from each other and give them supervised time together; shorter periods that keep increasing in duration as they are getting used to each other.

Mishka was one when Katrina brought six-month-old Niles into the household. Their guardians, Brenda and Katrina, thought Mishka needed a playmate. The trouble initially was that Mishka was not happy at all with the new addition.

Mishka was a quiet cat. He was extremely stressed and quit eating. He was so grumpy that they had to keep the cats separate.

Niles was happy-go-lucky and ready to play.

Brenda and Katrina were not getting anywhere with integrating the cats and were beside themselves with stress, concerned they were going to have to rehome Niles. That is when they called me to help.

Mishka would not eat when Niles was near and would hiss if Niles came near him. Once I explained to Mishka that Niles was there for him, he softened. He accepted Niles more and more. They went from being out only a short amount of supervised time together to being able to be together unsupervised all the time.

Initially, Mishka knew how to play with his human guardians and did not know how to play with another cat. Niles would keep trying to engage with Mishka, and Mishka did not want anything to do with Niles. Now Mishka and Niles play and tumble together, eat together, and snuggle together. Mishka has come full circle.

Sometimes Mishka initiates play, and Niles is not in the mood. Brenda and Katrina are immensely happy cat guardians.

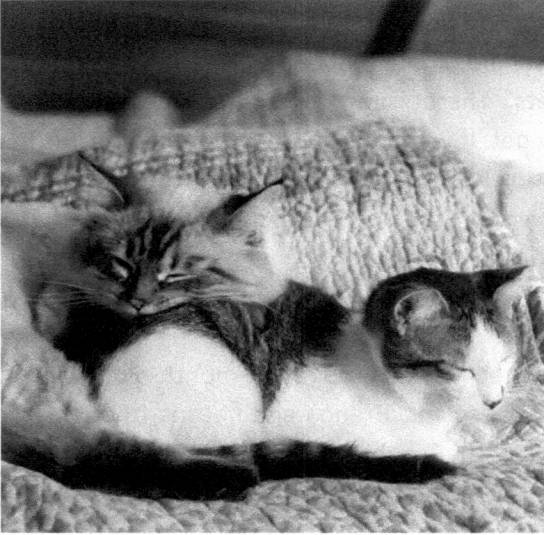

Mishka and Niles—photo submitted by Katrina Briggs

"Huge milestone here. Thanks to Vicki Draper and her fantastic holistic and intuitive skills, these two are now playing and getting along.

It's been amazing to watch this happen, and now they are cuddled up together.

We are beyond grateful and excited!"

—Brenda Reiss, Issaquah, WA

Preparing for a New Home

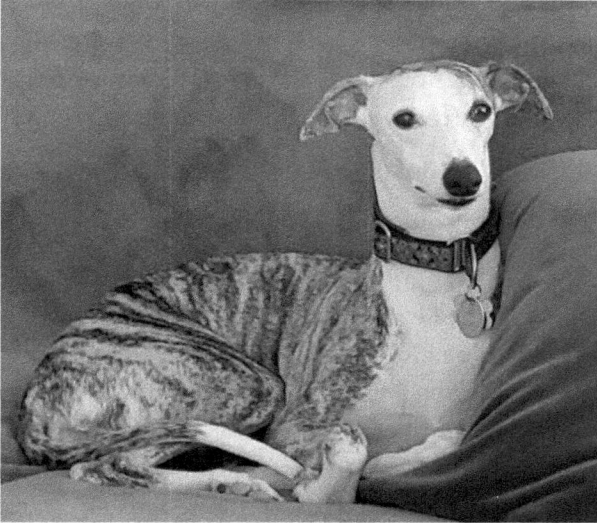

Farrah – photo submitted by Sheri Mortko

Just as I communicated and prepared Spirit and Sapphire for their new home with Miranda and me, Farrah received this treatment too.

Sheri is a long-time client who was between dogs. Before Farrah, a six-year-old Whippet, came home to Sheri's, we had a communication session to prepare Farrah for her new home and new life with Sheri and Rob.

Farrah was a breeding dog. She was used to being put in her crate often and not given much loving companion attention. Some show dogs are treated like parts of the family too, but not all of them. Some are treated as breeding and show dogs as their only purpose, period.

In Farrah's case, she was coming from a strictly breeding/show dog environment to a loving pet home environment. Sheri is a conscientious pet guardian and wants to honor her pet's wishes.

We connected with Farrah, helping her process the transition of leaving her pups and going to her new forever home. We blessed her and helped her understand that her puppies were going to their safe loving places too. One particular puppy of hers was highly sensitive, and Farrah wanted extra protections around her, so we did that.

We established that Farrah wanted to ride in the back seat of the car on the way to her new home.

We gave Farrah a "virtual tour" of her new home, by showing her the space energetically before they arrived. Farrah would not go in the kitchen because she was not allowed in the kitchen where she came from. I showed her that this was allowed in her new home. She was not allowed on the couch where she came from, so I showed her she was invited to be on the couch with snuggles. Also, she was not allowed on the bed where she came from. She ate, slept, and lived mostly in her crate. Farrah was invited to sleep on the bed in her new home if that was her choice.

I showed her she was going to her new home with new rules.

I received a photo of her first day at her new home where she had tried out her new cave bed, dog bed, the couch, and the guardian's bed, getting acclimated to her new home. I saw photos of her snuggling both of her guardians. The prep session really allowed this opening and freedom for her to integrate so easily and nicely into her new home.

We also shifted the energy of the meaning of her crate. Up until her new home, the crate was where she was put to get her out of the way. It was also, where she slept and ate and spent a lot of time, while another dog received loving attention and was allowed to roam free. Farrah was clear that she wanted a new crate, not the one from her previous home. Her new crate in her new home became her Light Palace. And she feels like a Princess. (These were Farrah's descriptions.)

She got used to being on the couch, and during her session, she energetically laid her head on Sheri's lap. Such love flowed through. It brought tears to my eyes. She was getting used to being shown and given love and affection.

Farrah was not used to playing with toys. Sheri and Farrah get to explore and find what she likes. This is a new adventure for both of them.

Forever Home

Forever home is a powerful tool, especially for animals being rehomed or rescued.

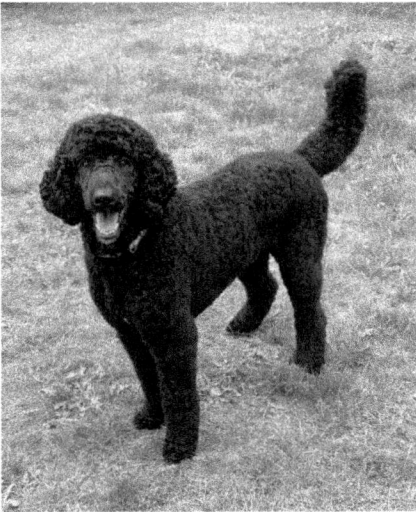

Rocky—photo submitted by Heidi Jellerson

Rocky, a ten-month-old labradoodle, was nervous, unsettled, confused, and sad. His previous guardian was crying when she dropped Rocky off to his new home with Heidi. Rocky did not know why he was at Heidi's. He was confused about what was happening. He would not eat much. He did not know if his prior guardian was coming back, and he carried that confusion and sadness when I met him.

Rocky's prior guardian and Heidi both knew this was Rocky's new home, but Rocky was still confused.

I started talking to Rocky about the heavy sadness he was carrying. He was open to letting it go, and he released it. His sadness turned out to be his prior guardian's sadness that he was carrying from when she dropped him off.

Rocky liked Heidi and liked being with her. During his session, as soon as he understood he was staying with Heidi, and he was in his forever home, that cleared his confusion. He knew what was happening, and he immediately started eating.

Riley, a young labradoodle dog, had severe separation anxiety. When Saleena, her guardian, would leave her to run errands, Riley chewed so hard on the metal of the crate that she bled. During her session, Riley paced around the room and would not settle down. As soon as I shared the fact that she was in her forever home and it resonated with her, Riley settled and laid down with a big plop. Riley was so relieved, and so was Saleena. It was clear to Saleena that Riley had experienced a big calming shift. There was no more blood when Riley was left in her crate.

Healthy Food

Health and wellness start with healthy food.

If you read food labels for your own food, then you know the importance of reading the food labels for your pet's food too. As with food for humans, the same goes for animals. Eating natural and organic foods that are not processed are healthier.

Feeding your cats and dogs healthy food is important for their health. Investing in good quality food will also save on veterinarian bills when your pet is older.

Did you know your cat's and dog's poop will not smell when you are feeding your animal a raw food diet? It is because all the ingredients are natural, and animals process and digest the food easily. The stinkier your cat's and dog's poop, the less healthy the food is for them.

In my experience, cats on dry food diets are more likely to have kidney failure. Cats need moisture in their food.

More benefits of feeding your cats a raw diet is they do not have many hairballs and their fur does not become matted.

Did you know the type of food you feed your cat or dog could affect their behavior? This is another reason to feed good healthy food.

Treats Matter

This goes as much for treats you feed your pets as it does for good nutritious food. Choose treats that are one ingredient, such as freeze-dried chicken or salmon, duck hearts. Investing in your pet's health now saves you stress and more veterinarian bills later.

Changing Your Pet's Food

When you change your cat or dog's food, it is important to wean them with a process rather than going cold turkey.

Here is what Shelley Knowles, Nutrition Specialist at Natural Pet Pantry in Kirkland, WA has to share:

Dogs

How to transition from kibble to stew (cooked at low temperature to preserve nutrients) or raw food depends on the age. With a young dog, the transition goes more smoothly; an older can be more challenging.

There are two ways to transition:

1. Feed nothing but a raw, fermented goat's milk diet for a couple of days to cleanse out their system and reseed the gut with good probiotics, prebiotics, and enzymes before introducing the new food. Then start introducing the new food, increasing the amount of food and decreasing the goat's milk. As long as things are going well, then you completely transition over. You can get this at Natural Pet Pantry, Kirkland, WA, Whole Cat & Kaboodle, Redmond, WA, at holistic, natural pet stores, and some natural grocery stores.

2. Add goat's milk to the current food you are feeding your dog, along with a little of the new food. Gradually increase the amount of the new food and decrease the amount of the original food until you are transitioned over fully to the new food.

Goat's milk has healthy, good bacteria, which your dog needs. If the dog has been eating highly processed food, they will not have all the good bacteria they need for healthy digestion. The goat's milk helps with making the healthy food transition.

Cats

You can do the same transition process of food for cats as for dogs, if your cat is accepting.

Some cats are more finicky and may not eat the goat's milk. Some cats will take right away to raw food, and others will not. There are two ways to transition to a raw food diet.

1. If your cat likes the goat's milk as described in the Dog section above, use it.

2. If your cat likes the raw food, add a small amount to their current food. Gradually increase the amount of the new food and decrease the amount of the original food until you are transitioned over fully to the new food.

Note: Some cats may take months before they will even taste the raw food or the new food. Patience is required for this process.

Tips for supporting your finicky cat in the healthy food transition:

1. Let them go past when they normally eat to get extra hungry before offering food.

2. Play with your cats to get their hunting instincts all fired up before feeding time.

3. For some cats, the problem is texture, so you can try:

    a. Adding warm water

    b. Putting it in a blender with water to make it a finer liquid

    c. Keeping it chunky, as some cats like it that way

4. For some cats, the problem is temperature, so you can try:

    a. Pan sear boneless food to warm it up and get the smells going

    b. Start out cooking the food (only if boneless), then gradually cook it less until you are serving it raw

5. Cats are creatures of habit, so change the location of where you feed them. When you put the food in a new location, they might be more curious about it, and they might try it.

6. Place a little dab of raw food on top of their current food. Cats may eat around it for months, and then finally, they eat the raw food.

Patience may be required for converting your cat.

When feeding good quality, healthy food such as a raw diet, your pets will eat less, their poop is firmer, and it does not have much smell.

During the food transition process, a detox process happens. If symptoms such as diarrhea and constipation occur as part of the detox, use the tools in Chapter 5: Common Issues Support to support your pet making the food transition more smoothly.

Play is Important

When you play with your cat, be sure to give them a treat or feed them afterward to reward them for their "kill" to emulate nature.

I like playing with Spirit and Sapphire in the morning. It is a fun way to start our day together, and then we have our breakfasts. We will also play before bedtime, so they get a treat after they have hunted the toy(s).

When you are playing with your dog, have healthy treats to reward your dog's good behavior.

Cat Litter Matters

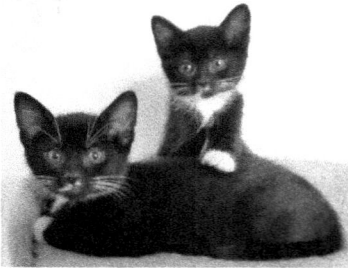

Wes and Maisy

Wes, a twelve-week-old kitten, was not playful and full of energy, which is not natural for a young kitten. Wes' guardians contacted me to see if I could help. During Wes' healing session, I discovered that he was reacting to the litter he was using. It was highly scented, and this was taxing his young body. We cleared his system and rebalanced him. The guardians immediately changed his litter, and he was back to being a normal, perky, into-everything kitten.

Cats, because it is in their nature to cover their pee and poop, are easily litter trained. You show them where the litter box is, and they will naturally do their business there (assuming they like the litter you are providing).

When selecting a litter, the type of litter matters for the health and life of your cat. Litter manufacturing has no regulations, so I encourage you to not price shop for litter. Using healthy litter may save you expensive veterinarian bills in the future.

For the safety of your cat, I recommend you use single-ingredient, natural, biodegradable cat litter such as pine, corn, soy, wheat, and grass.

Note: *Corn, soy, and wheat can be allergens to your cat. If your cat has signs of allergies, you will want to change the type of litter to the grass or pine type.*

Since cats dig in the litter to cover their pee and poop, any unhealthy dust such as clay or the sharp shards of silica may get into their lungs as they dig. Litter sticks to a cat's paws. The cat then grooms, so the litter is ingested. Over time, this may be extremely harmful with the unnatural litter such as clay, silica gel, and litter with added scents.

CHAPTER 2

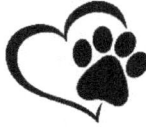

Preparing You for Healing Your Pet

THIS CHAPTER IS SO IMPORTANT that key information is repeated here from my first book, *Bridging True Love Connection & Healing Between You and Your Animals.* My intention is for you to gain knowledge and tools to support you to be calm, centered, and grounded for yourself, which also boosts your animal's well-being.

Even if you have read *Bridging True Love Connection & Healing Between You and Your Animals,* I encourage you to read this chapter, as some of it is presented in a new way. You will be reminded and discover a deepening of the information.

There are Five Key Energy Steps you will receive in this chapter.

Each of the Five Key Energy Steps corresponds with a Healing You Essence that make up the Energy Essentials Essence Package that work great for you and your animal.

If you are a person who likes the full experience, you are invited to order the Energy Essentials Essence Package to use daily as you incorporate the processes and techniques in this chapter:

HealingYourAnimal.com/PackagesForPeople.php

Step 1: Grounding

Grounding yourself is a key step in setting up a Healing Your Animal session with your animal.

The more grounded and calm you feel, the calmer and more grounded your animal will feel.

Now, you may be saying . . . Grounding?

That sounds woo-woo. Grounding is not woo-woo. People use that term when they do not understand.

You may know that I am a licensed animal massage therapist, certified animal acupressurist, craniosacral therapist, and Reiki Master/Teacher, and that I have a special gift for communicating and healing animals. What you may not know is that I also have a science background, with degrees in computer science, math, and physics.

So, what is grounding?

According to physics, the definition of grounding is the process of *removing* the excess charge on an object by means of the transfer of electrons between it and another object of substantial size.

In this case, *you* are the object with excess charge (anxiety, stress, hyperactivity) transferring these electrons to the Earth, which is the object of substantial size.

Recently, I taught eighth graders about the science behind grounding. We did a grounding exercise so they could experience it first-hand.

Interestingly, the children determined practical times when grounding would be helpful to them:

- When the teacher announces a pop quiz

- When they forgot to do their homework, which was due that day

- When they realized there was a test they forgot to study for

The eighth graders also shared their dog's behaviors that might indicate they were not grounded. For example, when their dogs:

- Spin around in circles

- Bark continuously

- Jump around too much

They got it! They understood!

I am confident you will too.

For you, an example of the positive charge is an excessively happy, over-the-top ecstatic person, charged with enthusiasm. An example of the negative charge is a nervous, fearful person, charged with fear and anxiety.

Grounding is great support, especially for multitaskers. When you have lots going on in your head and tons of energy, grounding will help you be clearer, more focused, and calmer in doing your multitasking, and you will be more efficient.

Grounding Exercise

- Stand up with your feet hip width apart.

- Close your eyes.

- Pretend you are a tree.

- Your body and legs are the trunk of the tree.

- Imagine you have big roots coming out of the soles of your feet.

- The roots go through the floor, through the top of the Earth, and deep into the Earth.

- Allow anything you are worried about to flow down your legs, into your roots, and out into the Earth.

Here are some ways for you to ground yourself:

a. Bring energy and focus down to your feet. Shuffle your feet, whether you are sitting or standing. Focus on moving your feet and feeling the connection to the ground or floor. This gets the flow of excess energy flowing down to the ground with attention on your feet. I find this technique easy because I can do it anywhere I am and at any time.

b. Take a walk. I recommend a 20-minute walk outside at a minimum. Walking also helps boost your immune system.

c. Walk barefoot on the Earth—in the grass or dirt (not on a sidewalk that is manmade). You can do this in the fallen leaves, dew, or snow to feel all seasons of the Earth.

d. Eat a meal. Food can be grounding. Beef, carrots, almonds, root vegetables, even chocolate are some common foods to help with grounding.

e. While sitting or standing, place the pinky finger of each hand on each of your creases in your legs where they meet your torso. Lightly place the palm of your hands on your lower body while your fingertips are pointing toward each other over your pubic bone. Gently close your eyes and notice what you feel. Hold this for 30 seconds to one minute (longer if you prefer).

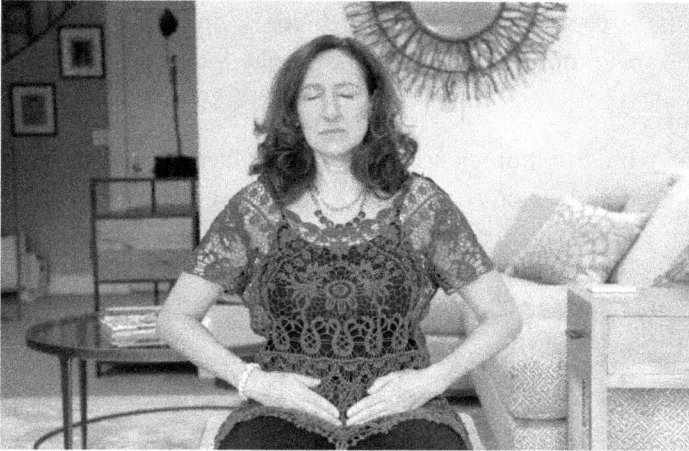

Photo by Jill Labberton, Jill Labberton Lifestyle Portraits

When you ground, you are not only calming yourself to feel safer and more secure, and you are helping your animal feel safer and more secure.

❧ *Your Essence Experience* ❧

For extra support, the Healing You **Ground** *essence is a natural, simple, effective, easy-to-use way to ground. Simply spray the essence three times in the surrounding air to receive grounding support.*

Step 2: Clearing You

You may be asking—What am I clearing? And why is this so important?

You have a physical body and an energy body. You know what your physical body is since you can see it, feel it, and touch it. You (and your animals) also have an energy body that most people cannot see or feel, but it is real. Your energy body does exist, and it needs attention and care to maintain the state of its health to support the health of your physical body. Did you know most disease starts in the energy body? When not cleared, the disease eventually goes into the physical body.

Regularly clearing your energy field is an important step in maintaining optimum health, not only for you, but for your animals too.

When you are not clearing, on some level, you are creating energetic clutter or chaos. In the same way that you can have physical clutter, you can have energetic clutter.

I know this to be true first-hand.

My own cat, Tasha, lived to be 19. She always slept with me and was always near me. She was what I call my "heart cat." We had a deeply close and special relationship. She was with me as I worked from home, and she would snuggle with me at night. She loved being with me. Any time I was not feeling well, she was by my side. When I let my life stresses build up and did not deal with them in a healthy way, she would quit sleeping with me and would throw up. I took her to the veterinarian each time. After getting her checked out by the veterinarian repeatedly, the veterinarian would find nothing wrong. I finally realized it was not something physical. I learned that as soon as I would clear myself and clear her, she would stay healthy, be by my side, and sleep with me again. She was a great teacher and a true barometer for me.

When you clear, you are introducing higher vibrations into your energy and your animal's energy field rather than contributing to and creating energetic clutter or chaos. You are bringing peaceful energy to yourself and your animal.

Taking a shower helps clear your energy field. So when you are in the shower, intend that your energy field is clearing as well as your physical body getting clean. Also, use Healing You *Clear* Essence to clear your energy field during the day.

I had a recent experience where I was feeling fatigued. I was on my way to lie down and rest when I decided to spray the Healing You *Clear* Essence first. As soon as I cleared, I was so full of energy. The heaviness lifted. It turns out I was tired because I was carrying around someone else's energy that was not mine. When it cleared, I was refreshed and revitalized.

This is one reason I recommend doing the five Key Energy Steps every day (and multiple times a day during times of high stress).

∾ *Your Essence Experience* ∾

Healing You **Clear** *essence is a natural, simple, effective, unscented, easy-to-use way to clear your energy field. Simply spray the essence three times in the surrounding air to receive clearing support and feel fresher. The* **Clear** *essence is a smokeless alternative to other clearing practices such as burning sage or palo santo wood, which can be harmful to people and animals with respiratory issues and compromised immune systems. And it does not leave the smell of smoke when clearing between clients in your healing practice, clearing your home, and clearing your hotel room when you travel.*

Step 3: Centering and Getting Present

Animals benefit from centering, just not in the same as humans. Animals are always present. As humans, we tend to be caught up in the past or the future and need reminders to be present and centered.

I like using animals as our teachers. And what do they do when they encounter something they need to release? They shake it off. For you, that is shaking off the worry about the past or the future and coming to the present moment.

Exercise 1:

Stand up, shake your arms, shake your legs, and shake your whole body. Check in and see how you feel.

Exercise 2:

Take a deep breath in, hold it for four seconds, let it out, and pause for four seconds. Take another deep breath in, hold it for four seconds, let it out, and pause for four seconds. Now for the power of three, take a deep breath in, hold it for four seconds, let it out, and pause for four seconds. Return to your normal breathing.

Take a moment, check in, and see how you feel. Can you feel a difference from just a moment ago before you took your three deep breaths? Is there more of an opening? More clarity? More awareness? More brightness? There is no right or wrong. Notice what it is for you.

Exercise 3:

Place your hands on your body one-and-a-half thumb widths below your navel. Hold for thirty seconds to one minute (or longer if you desire).

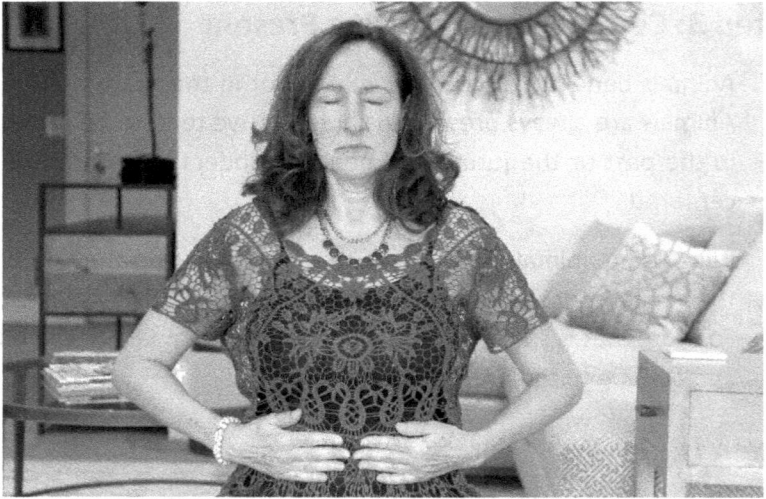

Photo by Jill Labberton, Jill Labberton Lifestyle Portraits

⤳ *Your Essence Experience* ⤳

*For extra support, the Healing You **Iceland Spar** essence is a natural, simple, effective, easy-to-use way to center. Simply spray the essence three times in the surrounding air to receive centering support. I invite you to take a deep breath in and let it out now after spraying the essence. I find this helps the essence integrate even more deeply.*

Step 4: Protection

You may be asking—What am I protecting? Why do I need it?

Your cats and dogs are most likely more energy-sensitive than you are. They are aware of energy that you might not be clued into. This sensitivity affects their behavior and how they feel.

Your energy field (or energy body, as some people call it) needs an energetic dusting, the same as your physical furniture in your house. This means clearing your energy field of what you have already picked up throughout your day.

Protection can help you and your animals not absorb energetic clutter as you go about your day.

What you are protecting yourself and your animals from is other people's energy, frustrations, anger, and other emotional stuff they are processing and dealing with.

This even goes for people when you are talking on the phone. Animals tune into what is going on. So the disagreement you may have with a family member or friend, your animals notice. Or if a friend calls and needs to vent, this is all part of energies coming into your energy field.

Why have protections? Just like you put on sunscreen to go out in the sun, you need to put on energetic protections to go into your day. It sets an energetic boundary, so that what is everyone else's is theirs and what is yours is yours. Therefore, no matter what you encounter, your energy field stays clean, and you feel clear and focused.

A common way to set up energy protection for yourself is to imagine a white light circling your body about an arm's width out from your body. It goes two feet above your head and two feet below your feet, forming a protective bubble of light around you.

Your protective bubble is semi permeable. It allows love and good in and out of your energy field, and keeps lower-level energies such as anger, depression, and anxiety out.

The protection helps you have more energy. When you are carrying around other's emotions and energies, it depletes your energy and vitality. This is the reason the Five Key Energy Steps are important, and also, why the Energy Essentials Essence Package supports you with optimum health and vitality.

❧ *Your Essence Experience* ❧

*For extra support, Healing You **Protection** essence is a natural, simple, effective, easy-to-use way to protect yourself from other people's energies and issues. Simply spray the essence three times in the surrounding air to receive protection support.*

*The **Protection** essence is one you may desire to use daily. When you do not sleep as well or you are not on full energy, **Protection** essence is an easy way to support your energy to stay strong and clear.*

Step 5: Expressing Gratitude

The more gratitude you have, the more things to be grateful for come to you in your life. To keep your vibrations high no matter what is going on in your life, have your first waking thoughts be:

Good morning! I am so grateful for _____ (whatever that is for you).

To support you throughout your day, I invite you to write down five things you are grateful for in your day. I also invite you to reflect on your gratitude list before going to bed. The more grateful you are for what you have, the more you will receive ease in your life. Giving focus to your gratitude list before you go to sleep will help you be in a better mood, which helps you sleep better.

๑ Your Essence Experience ๑

*For extra support, Healing You **Gratitude** essence is a natural, simple, effective, easy-to-use way to share gratitude. Simply spray the essence three times in the surrounding air to express gratitude to the Universe, opening ways for abundance and prosperity to flow back to you.*

If this feels like a lot of new information to you, it is ok. Becoming aware and being open to this information is a start. This is a process and journey. You have this book to come back to again and again to learn the material at different levels each time you read it. Start with where you are and keep growing at your pace.

Laura has a miniature labradoodle dog named Ginger. Laura is busy. She works a full-time job, is raising a daughter, and is very active in supporting her daughter's school by coordinating the school auction and more. At the end of this live training module, Laura's comment was, "I haven't felt this good in a long time."

This is why you are here. Helping your precious animal starts with helping yourself. Now you are ready to turn your attention to your animal.

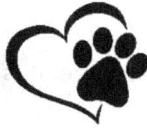

CHAPTER 3

Healing Session Protocol

THE INTENTION OF THIS CHAPTER is for you to learn the protocol of a healing session with your animal. The protocol consists of assessing, scanning, clearing, balancing, and integrating healing techniques with your animals for deeper healing and wellness care.

As you do more healing sessions with your animals, you will increase your assessing, scanning, clearing, balancing, and integrating abilities.

The healing session provides quality-bonding time together with your pet.

The first step in your animal's healing session is preparing you with the techniques from Chapter 2.

Setting Intentions

The second step is setting an intention for your pet's healing session. Intentions are visualizing or imagining your desired outcome.

Setting intentions is key in working with energy and healing sessions. You are sending a request to the Universe and allowing it to respond to you with what you desire.

When I use the word Universe, it is interchangeable with the term you use for your spiritual source. It is what some call God, Source, Universe, Higher Self, Buddha, or Guardian Angel. So whatever that is for you, please use it in place of the word Universe.

State your intention silently in your mind or aloud what you desire from your pet's healing session. It can be as simple as, "My intention is to provide care to my highest healing ability and for <insert your pet's name> to receive his/her highest healing good during our session."

If you have a more specific intention, state it.

Assessing

The third step is assessing and scanning to know what is going on with your animal's physical and energy bodies. Then you can do an integrating and closing of the healing session.

When you are assessing your cat or your dog, you are observing their health and demeanor to know whether they feel good or do not feel good.

The importance of assessing is it is a good preventative care practice. You will be able to find and detect issues earlier versus later to get your animal checked out by your veterinarian. Getting support faster makes it easier and quicker for your animal to heal. An example is finding a lump or a tender spot that is staying tender.

Assessing takes on three components, observation, scanning, and palpation.

Observation Assessing

Observe your pet's gait

- Is your pet walking normally?

- Is your pet holding his/her head up and straight?

- Is your pet walking evenly on both right and left sides?

- Is your pet limping?

- Is your pet walking slower than normal?

- Is your pet not jumping on places he/she usually does?

- Is your pet having more trouble getting up?

Observe your pet's eyes

Take note of your cat's or your dog's eyes. Are they bright and engaging? Or are they dull or lack spark, or appear listless?

The eyes are the windows of the soul and tell you about how your animal is feeling.

Observe your pet's gums

Pay attention to the gum color. A nice, healthy pink is a sign of good circulation. If you observe any bluish tint, get your pet to the veterinarian for oxygen and immediate care.

Observe your pet's coat

Pay attention to the quality of your pet's coat. Is it soft, shiny, and silky smooth? These are qualities of a healthy coat. Or is it dull or coarse, do you see white flakes and oil, or bare spots on his/her coat? These qualities suggest something is a little off in your animal. It could be something simple, such as a shift in your animal's diet, or it could be an indication of something more serious to have checked out by a professional.

Observe your animal's body language

Cats and dogs have multiple ways of communicating with you. The key is being open to receiving this information. They use their eyes, ears, mouth, tail, and body posture to communicate.

This site has body language charts and meanings for both cats and dogs:

bustersvision.org/animal-behavior-training/

They also communicate with pictures, feelings, taste, smell, and hearing. I am not covering these in this book. For more information on these, check out my first book, *Bridging True Love Connection & Healing Between You and Your Animals.*

Energy Assessment by Scanning

There is more to your animal (and you) than just the physical body. Your animal has an energy body that needs addressing for optimal health.

Did you know that most issues start in the energy field and have usually been there a while before they go into the physical body?

Therefore, regularly clearing your energy and your animal's energy field is important. You learned some clearing techniques for you earlier. Now, let us learn how to clear your animal's energy field.

For animals, it is important to daily clear their emotional and energy body to keep the physical body healthy.

I am teaching you how to clear you and your animal for daily wellness and maintenance. I also recommend a professional clearing for you and your animal on a regular basis. The professional is objective and sees the whole picture that you cannot see, as you are too close to your issues and too involved with your animals.

Our animals take on our issues. They do it because they are constantly in our environment, and they care about us. This is another reason it is good to do daily clearing techniques and have professional maintenance support on a regular basis.

My client, Kim, had two eleven-month-old puppies, Biscuit and Brulee, that were receiving wellness sessions. In one session, I noticed Biscuit had right hip energy that needed clearing. I thought maybe he tweaked it playing until I worked with Brulee. When I was working with Brulee, she also had right hip issues showing up to clear. Now, this was unusual for both puppies to have the same issue showing up at the same time. That is when I looked to Kim and asked, "Are you having right hip pain?" She said, "Oh yes, it has been acting up and is really bothering me." Biscuit and Brulee were "helping" Kim with her pain, and it was getting stuck in their bodies.

It is common for our animals to take on our "stuff." It is important for us to stay as healthy as possible and to do regular wellness clearing, centering, and protection.

Because we are close to our animals, it is important to stay as neutral as possible with no attachment when working with our animals for the best results. Let go of any agenda. Let go of what you know, so you are open to the experience and the information you receive.

For the purposes of this section, we will be working with the energy (etheric) body for scanning two to four inches off the animal's body.

The conditions of the energy body affect the visible physical body.

If the energy body by any means is affected, disturbed, or damaged, the visible physical body will also be affected.

The energy body is real, even though we cannot see it. You may have had an experience where something was getting close to you, and you could feel it, even though it was not touching you. That was your energy body giving you information.

Animals sense this very clearly.

The energy body is where the chakras flow and support you and your physical body.

Before I "came out of the closet" with energy work, I had a woman bring her dog to me for a massage. When the word massage is used, generally people think of it as a hands-on session. As we were doing our intake, she mentioned she wanted to try massage; yet she was not sure how her dog would like it. Her dog was not comfortable being touched. I explained that I could help her dog and honor him by not touching him. I did his whole session two inches off his body, working in his energy field with his energy body. Her dog loved it. He was so relaxed and content. She came back for another session because she could clearly see it worked and helped her dog feel better.

We are so conditioned to need to see things and touch things for them to be real, so this is counterintuitive. But it is effective.

Note: *Anytime you are going to do clearing, scanning, or massaging, you need to put on your energetic protective gloves.*

Put on an imaginary energy protection glove on each hand up to your elbows, similar to putting on gloves to wash your dishes. Set an intention that it will protect you from taking on your animal's energy that you are scanning. At the end of scanning and working in a healing capacity with your animal, take off the imaginary gloves while washing your hands and lower arms up to your elbows in cold water for the energy to separate. This way, what is your animals is your animals; what is yours is yours, and the rest of the energy released during your energy healing session goes down the drain.

Energy Scanning Method

To scan the energy body, start at the head with your hands two to four inches above your animal's body. Slowly move your hand straight down his/her body from the head until you reach the tail. While you are scanning, feel what is going on under your hand.

When scanning, you are listening with your hand and gathering information. The effect of scanning is that you are receiving information, and it also has a positive impact on your animal. A healing is occurring. It is not possible for you to move your hand with healing intent in your animal's energy field and not affect some change.

When scanning, it is important to flow down the outside of the front legs and up the inside of the front legs and flow down the outside of the back legs and up the inside of the back legs. This is the natural flow of the lymph system, keeping energy moving most effectively for the body to process.

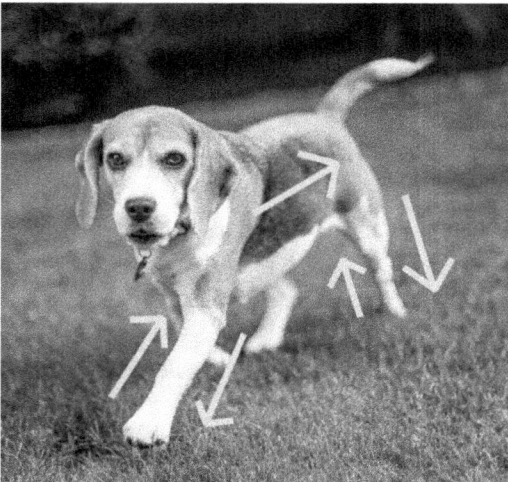

Effleurage Scan

After you have gone down the back from head to tail, start scanning your cat or dog's shoulders, down the outside of the leg to the paw, up the inside of his/her leg to the chest. (Do this on both sides. The order can be dependent on how your animal is lying, sitting, or standing. For example, finish scanning one side of the body if lying on one side before having them roll over to do the other side.)

Scan your cat's or dog's side. If they roll over here and present their belly, scan the underneath side of the body.

Scan the hips and down the outside of the leg to the paw, and up the inside of the leg.

Scan the jaws, throat, chest, rib cage, belly, and lower belly.

Do this until your whole cat or dog has been scanned.

Notice in particular what is going on in your hands

- Do you feel a sensation in your hands?
- Is the sensation hot, warm, or cold?
- Does the energy want to pull (suck) your hand down to the body?
- Does the energy want to push you out away from the body?
- Does it feel flowing, or does it feel stuck?
- Does it feel "sticky"?
- Notice the quality of energy as you scan

Notice what your cat or dog's body is doing

- Is your cat or dog wiggling when you scan a certain spot?
- Does your animal let out a sigh as you pass over a certain spot?
- Does your cat or dog start panting when you are on a particular spot?
- Are your cat's or dog's eyes widening or alert?
- Are your cat's or dog's eyes relaxing or closing?

Take notice of all this information you are receiving about your pet.

Physical Assessment by Palpation

In a healing session, and this includes when you are assessing, your animal may direct their session by rolling over and presenting the part of their body they want you to work with first before going on to another part. Animals have an innate connection of knowing with their body, and they listen to it.

I invite you to be mindful. Your animal may look to you like they are goofing off; however, they are engaging and giving you information. This is a new way for you to be with your animal, and there are subtleties in the information they provide.

A massage and healing session with your cat or dog is not the same as it is for you. For your massage, you lie on your front; your backside is massaged. You flip over, and then your front side is massaged without moving around. It is common for your animal to move around during the healing session. Be open, non-attached to an agenda of your assessment, and trust your animal. Your animal gives you a lot of nonverbal information. It is important for you to slow down and notice.

Assessing Your Pet's Physical Body

As a licensed animal massage therapist, I love to teach massage techniques.

There are some things to know first.

If your animal has an injury that has occurred within the last 48 hours, stop here. Do not do the assessment or effleurage. The injury is classified as acute. Go to Chapter 7 Pain Management and Aging Animals, to learn about Passive Touch.

If the injury is more than 48 hours old, it is safe to do the assessment using the massage techniques and then use the Wellness Protocol in Chapter 3.

Benefits of massage

- Increases your pet's relaxation

- Reduces stress

- Promotes wellness by assisting muscle tone, increasing flexibility, and improves circulation. Improving circulation is a catalyst to recovery after injury or after surgery.

  When I was volunteering at the Humane Society, one puppy named Michelle was so terrified that she was totally frozen in fear. She could not walk. As I was massaging her, she did start to relax a little. She was stretching her legs out more, yet not enough to walk. The muscles in her belly went from exceedingly taut to softer and more supple. When I came back the next week and asked about Michelle, she had been spayed. I was so grateful she had her massage beforehand so she had more relaxed muscles, as it would have taken overly tight muscles longer to heal after her spay surgery.

- Helps maintain energy and supports the immune system

- Provides information as a valuable diagnostic tool

- Enhances the bond between guardian and animal

- Accustoms your pet to being handled

In preparing to do a massage with your animal, there are times when it is not recommended or advised to give your cat or dog a massage, and those are called contraindications.

Contraindications to massage (when not to give your cat or dog a massage):

Physical circumstances:

- Do not work on or over the spine.

- Do not work on an open wound.

- Do not massage your cat or dog with a fever.

- Do not massage your cat or dog that is in shock.

- Do not massage a lump.

- Do not massage to a skin infection.

- Do not massage stings and bites.

- Do not massage acute inflammation (swollen, hot, red).

- Do not massage just after your pet has eaten. Wait three to four hours before massaging your pet.

- Do not massage if your pet is pregnant. Wait until after she delivers her litter.

- Do not massage your animal with cancer without veterinarian's consent.

- When in doubt, ask your veterinarian.

Non-physical circumstances:

- Do not massage when you are not mentally prepared (Angry, impatient, distracted, etc.).

- Do not massage if the animal tells you no.

  How do you know your animal is saying "NO?" (Just like you sometimes are not in the mood to be touched and want to be left alone, your animal has these moods too. It is important to honor them.) Your animal is:

o Shying away, moving away, or trying to get away from you

o Looking away, not engaging

Cats may show these signs:

o Tail flicking back and forth, the harder the flick, the more upset the cat is

o Ears are pulled back

o Hissing

o Growling

Dogs may show these signs:

o Ears back

o Head tucked avoiding you

o Growling

o Baring teeth

Massage is not a substitute for the medical advice of a veterinarian. A veterinarian should be consulted regularly, especially if any symptoms, which may require diagnosis or medical treatment, are present.

Now that you have determined it is safe to start massage and physical touch with your animal, it is time to learn effleurage.

Effleurage

A great technique to scan and assess your dog's or cat's physical body and warm up the muscles and tissues for a massage is a massage stroke called effleurage.

A French word meaning, "to skim" or "to touch lightly on," it is used in Swedish massage to warm up the muscles.

Effleurage is a light-gliding stroke with varying degrees of pressure (looks much like petting). The main difference between effleurage and petting is intent and a designated pattern flow. The purpose of all effleurage strokes is to "open" tissue by encouraging circulation. It moves the venous blood and lymphatic fluid. Strokes generally follow the coat and move toward the heart. Initial strokes are the weight of a nickel. Repeating the movement allows deeper penetration without increasing pressure.

I encourage you to do three passes with the effleurage stroke.

1. The first pass is starting to warm up the tissue, muscles, circulation, and lymph. It also is a chance for you to discover what is going on with your pet's body.

2. The purpose of the second pass is to open the tissue, muscles, circulation, and lymph even more. A second pass goes deeper without deeper pressure. It helps whatever issues that might have shown up in the first pass to receive healing and move on out.

3. The purpose of the third pass is to smooth out what has been opened and has been processing in your pet's body the first two passes. Issues that are not deep will generally clear by the third pass, making this a good wellness care technique.

If there are still issues after the third pass of effleurage, then your animal's body needs deeper techniques for their healing. That is a good indication it is time for a professional session.

When doing effleurage, gently rub with light pressure (the weight of a nickel) where your hand is softly engaging your cat's or dog's body.

Using both hands, start at the head, and rub down the head, one hand going to each shoulder and going **down the outside** of the front **leg**, down to the paws, **going up the inside** of the front **leg**, and coming up to the shoulders. Staying a little off to each side of the spine, rub your hands down the back on the side of the body to the hips. Now take your hands and rub them **down the outside** of the hind legs, to the paws and **up the inside** of their hind legs back to the hip and off the hind end to the tail, gently rubbing the tail to its tip and removing your hands.

Notice in particular what is going on under your hands:

- Is the quality of the muscle hard or soft?

- Is the area of the body hot, warm, or cold?

- Does the area or the muscle feel hollow, sinking in, empty or full, hard, protruding?

- Does the sensation under your hand feel flowing, or does it feel heavy, sluggish, or stuck?

Notice what your cat's or dog's body is doing:

- Are there muscle spasms or twitches?

  Muscle spasm is when you touch a place and the fur crawls. It looks like ripples on parts of your animal's body. This means something is out of balance and putting strain on the muscles.

  A twitch is a smaller spasm that happens quickly. You may see it clearly. If you catch it out of the corner of your eye, you may wonder if it really happened.

- Is your cat or dog wiggling when you touch a certain spot?

  If your animal is moving or wiggling, you may think they are goofing off and being silly when they are really responding to where you have touched their body. The best way to know if this is the case is to repeat touching the same area to see if there is a reaction again.

- Does your cat or dog release a sigh as you rub over a certain spot?

When your animal lets out a big sigh, there is tension that is released. This is a sign your animal is responding and relaxing.

Your cat or dog may settle after a sigh.

- Does your cat or dog start panting when you are on a spot?

Just as when you get a massage and a sore spot is being worked out, your massage therapist will say to breathe, take a deep breath in and out to help it move on through. This is what your animal is doing when panting during a session where there is a sore spot. You will notice the panting subside once the soreness has been reduced.

- Are your animal's eyes widening?

Your animal's eyes widening is a sign you are nearing or on a sensitive spot.

- Are your animal's eyes relaxing or closing?

Pay attention to your animal's eyes during the healing session. You will notice them softening as they relax. Endorphins release during your animal's massage the same way they do for your massage.

The more you do effleurage, the more you will tune your hands to feel what is going on under them. You will start to feel some sensations. Pay attention to how you receive the information. Be mindful and notice what is happening under your hands as you assess with effleurage.

You will form a baseline with your animal. You will know what is normal and what is not. This helps you get needed care as soon as possible for your precious animal.

Assessing Pain

As I was assessing and scanning Solomon, a seven-year-old Japanese and Neapolitan mastiff, pit bull breed, as soon as I got past his shoulders, he would roll over on his back and start wiggling on the ground. He would come back, I would start assessing again, get to the same spot behind his shoulders, and he would roll on his back and start wiggling again. He was a regular client. He had never had this behavior before during an assessment. He was telling me his mid-back was tight. Once we got the tension worked out, he did not roll over and wiggle anymore. To a bystander, it could have looked like Solomon was just playing around. When in fact, he was sharing information that his back was tight.

In another session, Solomon would not lay with his hind right leg on top. He would continue to lie on it even after having him get up, walk around, and lie back down. When something like this happens, it is the time to be curious. I wondered if his left or right hind leg and/or hip was having an issue or if he was in pain. I started working with his hind right leg where I could reach it with him lying on it. He was holding it tight against his body. As I was working his lower right leg, he started to relax his leg and stretch it out. This told me it is his right hind leg having the issue. Having Solomon stand and lie down again, he then presented his right hind end on top by lying on his left side. I was able to fully support his right hind quarters.

Regularly doing a healing session helps catch issues quickly.

Sanja, a German shepherd, was a regular client. One day, when I was massaging Sanja, she would squeal when I lightly touched the left side of her upper belly. This was not normal. I could tell it was not a muscular issue, so I advised Sanja's guardian to take her to the veterinarian.

The veterinarian was amazed, saying usually he did not get cases of pancreatitis until it had progressed much further. Catching it early, Sanja was able to get the medical support she needed and quickly heal.

Early detection is key in supporting your animal with optimum health.

Assessing Lumps

When you discover a lump, I highly encourage you to get it checked out by your veterinarian. Some cancers are slow growing, some are excessively aggressive, and some lumps are benign (non-cancerous). The only way to know is by visiting your veterinarian.

In the case of a lump, early detection can be crucial. This was the case for Sophie, a four-year-old miniature poodle. Claire, Sophie's guardian, discovered a small lump. She immediately took Sophie to the veterinarian. It was cancer. Catching it early helped Sophie get the treatment started to keep the cancer from spreading.

I was also able to do an early assessment with Tuck, an 18-year-old cat, who is a regular client that receives massages every three weeks. Even when Cathy, Tuck's guardian, was out of state, Tuck was getting her regular healing sessions. I discovered a lump behind Tuck's ear. Tuck was able to get into the veterinarian and get the lump removed. The biopsy came back as cancer, and all of the cancer was removed. Whew!

This is the importance of regular sessions. Had Cathy waited until she returned for Tuck's sessions, I would not have caught it so early.

Now that you have assessed, scanned, and warmed up your animal's physical body with the effleurage, we are going into the healing portion of your animal's healing session.

Clearing

Clearing is different from scanning. When clearing, you are collecting the energy and releasing it.

Use what I like to call the "tip of nose to tip of tail" technique for clearing your animal.

Put on your energy protection gloves as you did earlier in this chapter.

Hold your hand two to four inches above your animal's body. Start with your hand over the nose and run your hand above your animal's body, down the centerline, all the way to the base of the tail. As you are doing this, envision collecting everything that is no longer needed from your animal's energy field into your hand as you pass from the nose, over the forehead, down the back of the head, over the shoulders, down the center of the back, over the hips, and out the base of the tail.

A quick review from science: According to the law of conservation of energy, energy can never be created or destroyed. Energy can only change forms.

Once you have completed this, imagine you are flicking the energy off into an imaginary, one-way energy recycle bin to remove it from your hand, with your glove still on. The intention is to let go of all of the energy no longer needed, what is ready to release, what isn't your animal's energy that he/she collected throughout the day. Visualize the released energy being transformed for where it is to go next.

The intention is that your animal's energy field is replenished with light, optimal health, healing, and high vibrational energies. Nature abhors a vacuum, so after you clear, it is important for you to replenish the area by visualizing it filled with light, optimal health, healing, and high vibrational energies.

↩ *Your Essence Experience* ↩

*Healing Your Animal **Clear** essence is a natural, simple, effective, unscented, easy-to-use way to clear your animal's energy field. Simply spray the essence three times in the air around your animal to receive clearing support and feel fresher.*

Balancing

When my daughter, Miranda, was in kindergarten, I helped organize a field trip for her class to the Northwest School of Animal Massage. We went to the barn to help the children learn about horses. When the instructor traced the bladder meridian on the horse to open the energy and balance the energy of the horse, even amid the class of excited kindergarten students, the opening and balancing energy was palpable. We could see it was calming to the horse.

Tracing the bladder meridian on cats and dogs works the same way, producing the same effects.

(For larger charts where the numbers are more visible, see the Resources section at the end of the book.)

Feline Bladder Meridian Chart ©2020

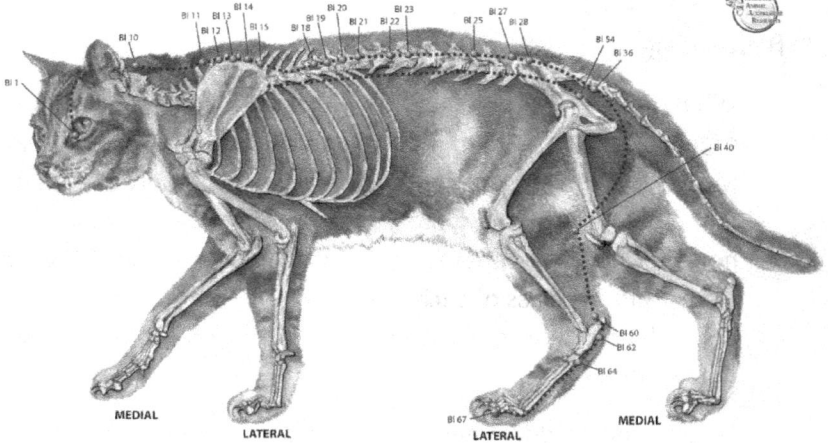

Canine Bladder Meridian Chart ©2020

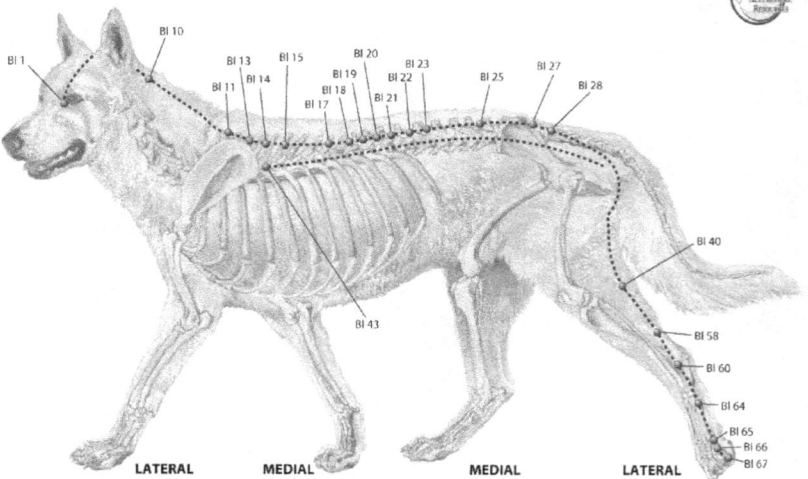

Acupressure Charts: Permission was granted by Nancy Zidonis and Amy Snow of Tallgrass Animal Acupressure Resources.

What makes the bladder meridian so powerful (in our animals and us) is there are acupoints on the bladder meridian parallel to the spine that associate, innervate, and run through each of the organs in the body. The importance of keeping the energy of these points in balance is that it promotes wellness.

Tracing the Bladder Meridian

As you are tracing the bladder meridian, pay attention to the information you are collecting and receiving, the sensations occurring, and your pet's reactions to your touch in certain areas.

Begin at the point on the inside of the eye at the bridge of the nose. Run your finger up and over the top of the head to the side of the midline, and down the neck.

At the shoulders, the meridian turns into two paths, emotional and physical.

We will focus on the physical path, which is about a finger width from each side of the spine. Depending on the size of your animal, the meridian may be slightly closer or further from the spine. (The emotional path runs another finger width or so from the spine.)

Follow the physical path over the tip of the shoulder blade.

Your finger will fall into a natural divot behind the tip of the shoulder blade. This is the start of the physical organ association of the bladder meridian. Follow the path down to the base of the tail, which ends the physical organ association of the urinary bladder meridian. Keep following the path down the midline of the back of the leg, at the knee/stifle, shift slightly to the outside of the hind leg down to behind the ankle and out the outside of the paw.

Notice what is going on under your fingers from your animal's shoulder blades to the base of the tail:

- Is the sensation hard or soft?
- Is the sensation hot, warm, or cold?
- Does it feel hollow, empty, or full, protruding?
- Does it feel flowing, or does it feel stuck?

Notice what your animal's body is doing:

- Are there muscle spasms?
- Is your cat or dog wiggling when you touch a certain spot?
- Is there a sigh as you rub over a certain spot?
- Does your cat or dog start panting when you are on a particular point?
- Is your cat's or dog's eyes relaxing or closing?

Now you have information from the first pass, and it is time to make a second pass.

- Notice if the sensations have stayed the same or changed.
- Notice if your pet's reactions are the same or different.
- Notice if your pet's reactions are in the same areas or if they are in different areas.
- Is your pet reacting more or less on the second pass?

The purpose of the first pass is opening the bladder meridian.

The purpose of the second pass is going deeper with opening and balancing the bladder meridian.

Now, make a third pass on the bladder meridian. Again, notice:

- What sensations are you feeling under your finger?

- Are your pet's reactions the same or different in the same areas?

- Are your pet's reactions different in different areas?

- Is your pet reacting more or less?

By the third pass, it is common for any reactions from your pet to clear, as you have moved blocked or stagnant energy out of the area, which relieves discomfort. And if an area has been overstimulated with excess energy, you have helped get the energy back into balance again, and relieving discomfort.

If, after the third pass, your pet is still reacting to a specific spot, you will know there is a deeper issue that needs to be addressed. That is a good indication it is time for a professional session.

Tracing the bladder meridian opens flow for the wellness of your pet throughout your animal's healing session.

ೞ Your Essence Experience ೞ

*For extra support, the Healing Your Animal **Iceland Spar** essence is a natural, effective, easy-to-use way to center. Simply spray the essence three times in the air around your animal to receive centering support.*

✦✦✦✦✦✦✦✦

Note: *Here you can insert additional techniques from the following chapters into your animal's healing session.*

✦✦✦✦✦✦✦✦

Integrating and Closing

All the work that has happened during your healing session needs time and space to integrate into your pet's body. We help this integration in the closing of each of your healing sessions with your pet.

- **Effleurage**—This is used for opening the body for a healing session. We also used it as an assessment tool. We will also close the healing session with effleurage. Now that you are aware of the bladder meridian, you see that the bladder meridian is worked during effleurage. For closing, make two passes of effleurage on your pet. Lighten your pressure on the second pass.

- **Final pass grounding**—This is the third pass of effleurage, done with an even lighter touch. As you rub the outsides of the front legs down the front paws, pause on the paws for three to five seconds. Continue up the inside of the front leg, along the side of the body, slowly down the hips and the back leg to the paw, pausing again at the back paw for three to five seconds. Continue up the inside of the leg and out the tail, lightly lifting your hands off the end of the tail.

- **Sweep the energy field**—This technique is where you start with your hands at the top of the head, four to six inches off the body, make a pass down the center above the body over the head, down the midline, and out above the tail. Flick the energy to the figurative recycle bin.

  Next, start with your hands four to six inches off the body on the left side above the face, move along the left side above the body from front to rear, and flick the energy after you pass the tip of the tail to the recycle bin.

  Repeat this on the right side above the body.

- Rub your hands together to disconnect the energy of the healing session.

- Thank your pet for the session.

- Thank your space for the session.

- Separate yourself from the healing session. Wash your hands in cold water up to your elbows while removing your energy gloves and allow all that is not yours or your animal's (what has been released in the session) to gently clear down the drain. The energy is being recycled for its next purpose. All energy that is yours is yours, clearly separated from the healing session. And all that is your animal's energy is your animal's.

❧ Your Essence Experience ❧

*For extra support, Healing Your Animal **Protection** essence is a natural, simple, effective, easy-to-use way to protect your animal from other people's and animal's energies and issues. Simply spray the essence three times in the air around your animal to benefit with protection support.*

Celebrate! You have received the healing session protocol. The techniques you will learn in the following chapters can be easily added to this protocol for maintaining optimum health with your pet for all stages of his/her life.

CHAPTER 4

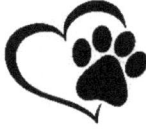

Wellness Techniques

THE INTENTION OF THIS CHAPTER is to build on the Healing Session Protocol to deepen wellness care for all stages: puppy/kitten, teen years, and aging animals.

Wellness Protocol

Regular healing sessions with the protocol from Chapter 3 done weekly provides the foundation of natural wellness care.

Additions to the Wellness Protocol

The techniques in the protocol warm up the tissue so you can now do some deeper work. Here are additional techniques to add to the protocol:

Chucking—Sections of muscle are pushed together and released; mostly used on the lower legs.

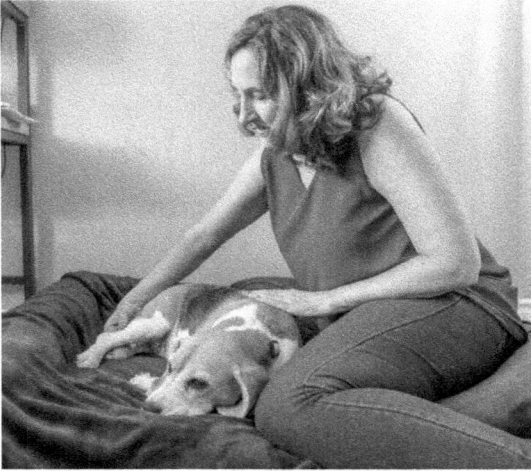

Chucking

Finger/Digital Circles—Using the pads of your fingertips, apply a light, circular motion. Use this technique around the shoulder blades, base of rib cage, around the hip bones, and parallel to the spine.

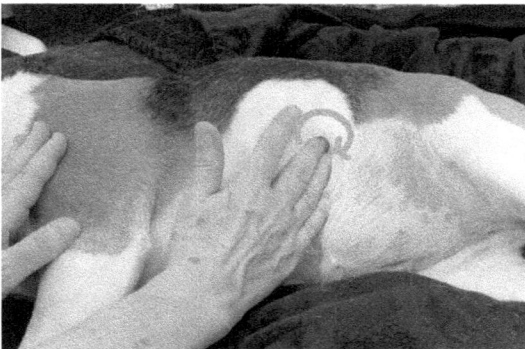

Digital Circles

Gliding—Use a deeper massage stroke, passing a finger or thumb along the length of a muscle or area. This is used primarily along the side of the spine and base of the rib cage.

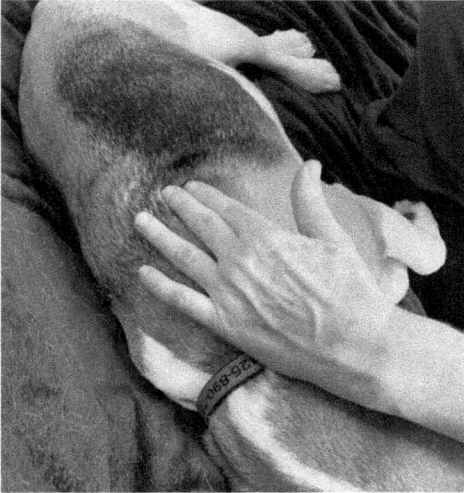

Gliding

Petrissage—Knead muscle (lifting and squeezing tissue) using the fingers and thumb.

For the neck area for cats and small dogs, use one hand, with your thumb on one side of the neck and index and middle fingers on the other side, and gently lift and squeeze the neck muscles.

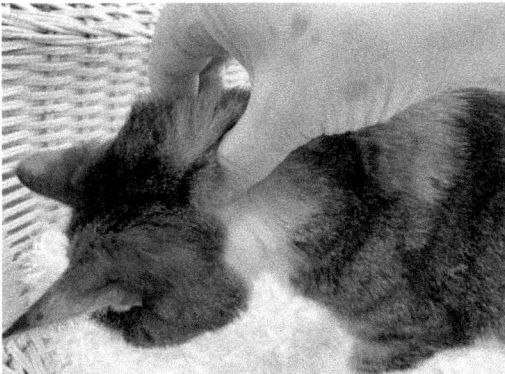

Cat Petrissage

For medium-size dogs, use one hand, with your thumb on one side of the neck and all four fingers on the other side, and gently lift and squeeze the neck muscles.

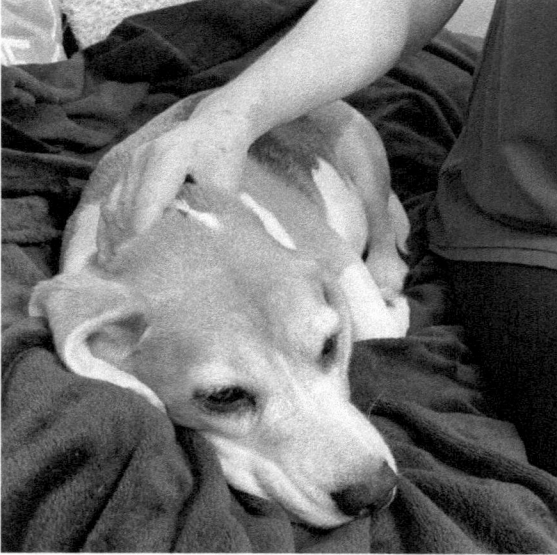

Dog Petrissage

For large and extra-large size dogs, use two hands, with one hand on each side of the neck, and gently lift and squeeze the neck muscles.

Raking—Use a cross-fiber stroke; cupped fingers are dragged across the ribs. Raking is a massage technique that is important because every step your four-legged friend takes impacts the muscles on all sides of their body. Raking uses your fingers to go between the ribs on both sides to keep your animal moving with ease and breathing easier. Depending on the size of your pet, your fingers may not literally fit between the ribs (for example, cats and small dogs).

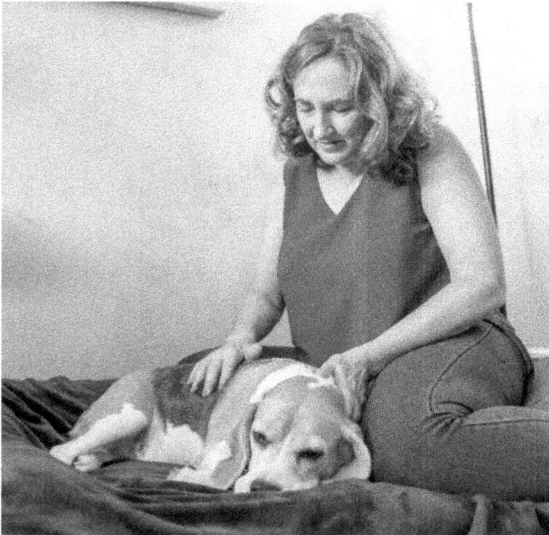

Raking

Start with your fingers a half-inch from the spine and stroke down both sides to the center of the chest. Do this for both sides.

Sifting—Gently grasp muscle fiber of the upper leg between your fingers and thumb. Fingers are on the inside of the upper leg and your thumb is on the outside of the upper leg. Move your fingers underneath, across the muscles to the outside edge. This technique is mostly used on the upper front and back legs. For smaller dogs, your fingers will support all the muscles in both the front and back upper legs. For medium and large dogs, you will need to do a pass on both sides of the upper legs to support all the muscles.

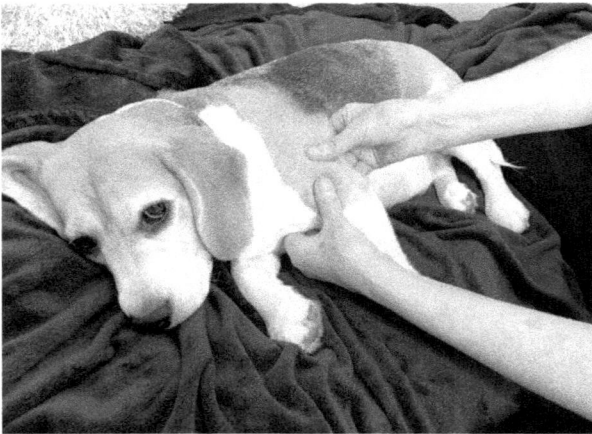

Sifting

Standalone Wellness Techniques

Some techniques can be used for wellness that do not require warming up the tissues first. Some of these you will recognize as the warm-up techniques from Chapter 3 in the healing session protocol.

Bladder Meridian

Tracing this meridian is a great wellness tool, as all the points associated with the organs are located on it. By tracing the bladder meridian, as you learned in Chapter 3, you are providing wellness by stimulating each of the organs for healthy flow. For instructions on how to trace the bladder meridian, refer to Chapter 3.

Ears

Rubbing your pet's ears stimulates acupressure points that map to the organs and systems in your pet's body, keeping your pet healthier. It is a simple wellness technique, and your pet will most likely enjoy it, no matter their age.

If you have an especially young kitten or puppy that is not eating, rubbing the ears will help stimulate the suckling response to help them eat. Their ears are tiny, so only gentle rubbing is needed with your index finger and thumb, one on the inside and the other on the outside of the ear.

I demonstrated this to a local animal board and training facility with a kitten less than a week old that would not eat. While massaging the kitten's ears, the kitten started moving and licking its lips, ready for food.

Massage and Effleurage

Using these simple and powerful techniques increases circulation, moves the lymph, and warms up the tissue. Effleurage is also a great tool for discovering what is happening in your pet's body.

Being familiar with your pet with regular effleurage helps you find any changes occurring in your pet's body, such as lumps, so you can quickly get the proper care when needed.

Effleurage also gets your animal used to being touched. It is helpful to massage their paws too, so that when veterinarian examination and nail trim time comes, it is not a big deal.

For instructions on how to do effleurage, see Chapter 3.

Puppies and kittens are wiggly and on the move, so you may need to make regular touch into a game. While one hand is doing the massage, the other hand is distracting them. Since they wiggle so much, you need to have patience and realize you are doing a good job and making a difference even though you have a moving target in your arms.

With puppies and kittens, the massage should be shorter. They are young, so their system (and attention span) can only tolerate shorter sessions of five to fifteen minutes, gradually increasing the time up to thirty minutes.

Puppies and kittens are very playful, rambunctious, and active. Most tumbles their bodies can recover from easily. There can be a time when they need professional help to relieve an issue before it turns into a bigger issue if gone unsupported.

An example is when a young animal takes a big jump and lands improperly. That can jam toes and put extra stress on the muscles that may go into spasm and not release on their own. These cause your puppy or kitten to start guarding the tender spot, impacting their gait so that they start walking unevenly. It may be slight, or it may be obvious. Either way, uneven walking puts extra stress on the body, and compensating muscles are overworked. When this happens, the body is out of alignment.

A wellness massage can tend to these muscles, and it is easier to heal when done soon after the incident. The longer an issue builds up, the longer it takes to heal.

It is common to think that puppies and kittens are young and do not need wellness care. That is not true.

Sapphire is an example of a kitten needing care that impacted her quality of life and mobility.

When she was a six-month-old kitten, she had trouble jumping on the counter. Spirit, her brother, had no problem. I would see her try and then fall.

Sapphire was not a lap kitten. Once she jumped off, she was done, and did not come back. And if she was brought back, she immediately jumped off again.

I was working on her back, and when I got to the tight muscles, she ran off the couch, paused, integrated what just happened, and miracles of all miracles, she jumped back onto the couch into my lap for more. She realized it was helping and wanted more.

Miranda and I were amazed. This was so out of character for Sapphire.

After doing massage with her, I took Sapphire to the veterinarian to get chiropractic support. The veterinarian thought Sapphire's eyes might be the issue, causing her not to gauge her jump correctly. This jumping and missing did impact her low back. With chiropractic support and doing massage with her, she was able to jump freely again.

Scout is an example of a puppy needing care that impacted his quality of life and mobility.

I was visiting with the family when Scout, a one-and-a-half-year-old Pomeranian puppy, got up from the couch, stretched both front legs and only his back left leg. Without palpating him, I did not know if there was an issue or not. Once I noticed this, I kept an eye out. I was wondering if it was a one-time thing or a repeatable pattern.

When it was repeated, I knew for sure something was up with his right hind leg.

When I palpated his right hind leg, he had tight muscles in his hock (the anatomical pronunciation for the animal's ankle joint). After relaxing the muscles, he stretched all four legs.

This was something better to catch earlier than have it continue as he got older and stiffer. Scout will now be able to move better longer in life.

Toes

Stimulating the toes and web of toes gets your pet used to grooming and having nails trimmed.

Ting Points—Stimulating the ting points is extra healthy, as this is where the yin and yang meridians meet. This helps keep a healthy flow of chi (Universal Life-Force Energy) through all the organs, since they are associated with the meridians.

The ting points are located on both the front and back paws.

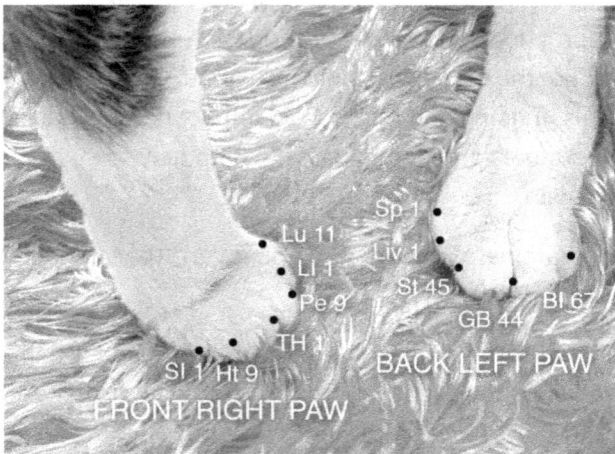

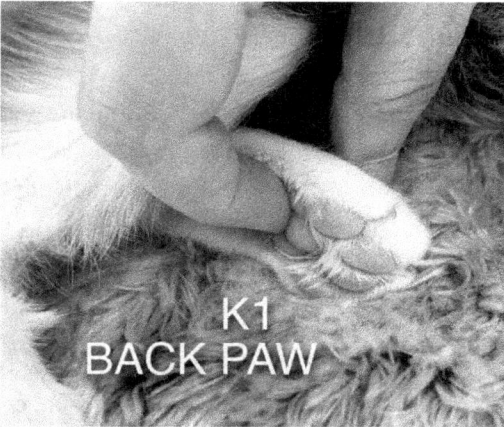

To stimulate the ting points, gently squeeze each toe at the base with the nail between your fingers.

Do this for all four paws. Remember to include the dewclaw. If the dewclaw has been removed, the bone is still there to stimulate. On the hind paws, gently stimulate below the pad in the middle of the paw.

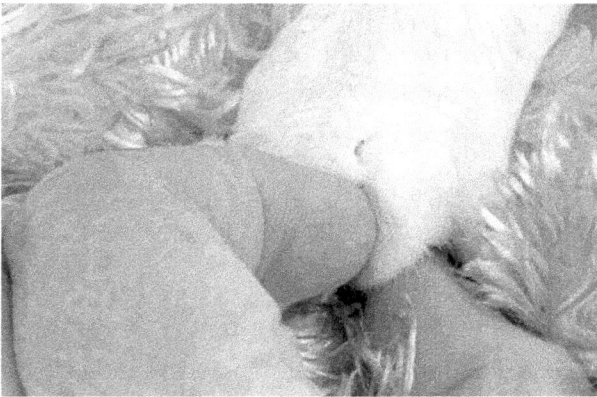

Ting Point Stimulation

Web of toes—Rubbing the web of your pet's paws helps them get used to their paws being touched and helps keep circulation and energy moving.

Aromatherapy

Aromatherapy and essential oils are all the rage. As a loving, responsible pet guardian, it is up to you to know that some essential oils are known to be toxic to your pet. Some are so toxic that one drop placed on them can put them into liver failure (especially cats). Cats are more sensitive to essential oils than dogs. Dogs are not as sensitive as cats, yet they do have sensitivities to be aware of.

NOTE: Aromatherapy and Healing You and Healing Your Animal Essences are not the same. Aromatherapy works through the olfactory system when you smell the oil. Essences are unscented and work through the parasympathetic nervous system when sprayed.

What is not taught and shared when you make oil purchases is that some aromatherapy is not healthy for cats, whether used topically or in air diffusers. Simply wearing the oils around pets can be toxic to them. Some oils are extremely toxic—one drop on your cat can cause death, and even breathing in some of the aroma from a diffuser in the air can cause death.

You may be using or be tempted to use some essential oils during the cold, flu, and now coronavirus season.

More products are adding essential oils to them, so the risk is getting even greater for your pets to be exposed to them. Since this information is not widely available, I want to educate you about this topic.

I have cats, I am scent sensitive, and I have a private practice working with pets, so I have not used many essential oils for my healing purposes, knowing I am keeping all of the animals I am around safe.

Even knowing the information for years that essential oils can be toxic to your pet (especially cats) and being extra careful, I fell into the trap of putting my cats in danger. Miranda, my daughter, had given me an essential oil and diffuser kit for my birthday. She knows I like relaxing and healing time after providing that for others. She did not know the oils could be toxic to our cats. I had opened the kit to let her know it was a thoughtful gift. I had a nasty cold, and I was having trouble breathing. I put eucalyptus oil into the diffuser to get some relief. As I was feeling better and better, I looked over at my cat, Spirit, who was hanging over the top shelf of the kitty stand, eyes glazed over, lethargic, and suffering from heavy breathing. I jumped up and immediately turned off the diffuser and opened the windows to clear the air. I then looked up essential oils toxic to cats. Eucalyptus was one of them. I immediately cleared out the oils, keeping only three out of the twelve-pack that are safe to use with cats in the household. I promptly educated Miranda too. Nowhere on the packaging was it listed that some of the oils are not safe for pets.

After 20 years of being careful, knowing some essential oils were toxic to cats, I put my cats in danger. I was not thinking clearly with the cold I had, and I did not have all the information. I did not realize diffusing the oils would be toxic. In fact, it is extremely toxic to diffuse essential oils. Since oil and water do not mix, the full effect of the oil is being spread into the room.

Now I know, and now you know.

Symptoms to look for in your pet when using aromatherapy and essential oils:

- Distress
- Heavy or very shallow breathing
- Shaking Excessively
- Drooling
- Squinting
- Rubbing their face

- Vocalization
- Vomiting
- Tremors
- Diarrhea

Essential Oils Toxic to Cats

Here are the lists with the most known toxicity for cats. When in doubt, do not use the essential oil. Not all veterinarians are educated on essential oils, so they may not be your best resource. Ask your veterinarian to see if they do know about it or consult with a certified aromatherapist before using any essential oils in your house and especially for your pet.

For cats, being exposed to the following essential oils can cause severe liver damage, seizures, liver failure, and even death.

- Eucalyptus oil
- Cinnamon oil
- Wintergreen oil
- Peppermint oil
- Sweet birch oil
- Tea tree oil
- Citrus oil includes lemon oil, orange oil, and tangerine oil.
- Clove oil

In researching the information for my podcast, *Animal Messages: What Your Animals Want You To Know* Episode 9: "Your Aromatherapy May Smell Good To You; Yet, It May Be Killing Me," I found a site that at first seemed reliable, but said eucalyptus oil was safe for cats and **that is not true**. Snopes agrees and has an article confirming eucalyptus is not safe to use around cats. Again, when in doubt, do not use the essential oil. In addition, talk with your veterinarian before buying and using products that contain essential oils.

Essential Oils Toxic to Dogs

Exposing dogs to the following essential oils can cause serious problems and even death.

- Cinnamon oil
- Pennyroyal oil
- Wintergreen oil
- Peppermint oil
- Sweet birch oil
- Tea tree oil
- Citrus oil such as lemon oil, lime oil, orange oil, or tangerine oil
- Pine oil

This list may not be fully comprehensive. Do not take chances. Stay away from blends and products that have one of these oils included. And when in doubt, do not use the essential oil. Not all veterinarians are educated on essential oils, so they may not be your best resource. Ask your veterinarian to see if they do know about it or consult with a certified aromatherapist before using any essential oils in your house and especially for your pet.

You have heard what not to do with aromatherapy with your cats and dogs, but there *are* times aromatherapy is good for your pets.

After doing the podcast about aromatherapy, I interviewed Joan Sorita, an aromatherapy expert, about how we can safely use this therapy with cats and dogs.

Here are some highlights of what Joan wants you to know:

- Lavender—Not all lavender essential oils are created equal.

    Not Safe: Lavender grossa, mainly grown on the coast, is not safe for animals.

    Safe: Lavender Augustifolia is a good one to use for animals.

- Get your essential oils from a reputable source in pure format. Some essential oils are not pure. Some are mixed with a carrier oil to dilute them. You may be paying the price for a full pure oil.

- Some companies mix lower-cost essential oils into higher-priced essential oils. You may be paying the price of the pure oil instead of the mixture oil.

- Some companies mix synthetic ingredients that can cause issues for you and your pet.

- Diffusing essential oils is extremely toxic to your pet.

Joan shares the safe way to use essential oils is to have your pet smell the oil. Your pet knows what their body needs. They will self-select the oil best for them.

If you are interested in more information about what is safe with aromatherapy for your pets and learn about some calming and physical aches support formulas, I invite you to listen to Episode 15 my podcast interview with Joan, "Learn Safe Aromatherapy For Your Cat And Dog." You will find it on the major podcast platforms.

Now you are ready to keep your pets safe with this information.

See the resource section for the Aromatherapy Top Supplier Sheet recommended by aromatherapy expert Joan Sorita.

Support *When Your Pet Is Taking an Antibiotic*

There may come a time when your pet needs to take an antibiotic. Just like with people, it is helpful to supplement with a probiotic to help balance the digestive area and keep it healthy.

There are two schools of thought when adding in the probiotic with an antibiotic.

1. Start the probiotic after you finish the antibiotics and use for two to four weeks.

2. Use the probiotics the same days as antibiotics, but at different times, and continue afterwards for a few weeks. If your pet's antibiotic is given one time per day, give the probiotic twelve hours later. If your pet's antibiotic is given twice per day, split the time between doses to give the probiotic.

I recommend discussing which option and dosage of probiotic is best for your pet with your veterinarian. They do not always remember to tell you to take the probiotic when taking antibiotics. However, in my experience, if I ask about it or have my clients ask about it, veterinarians have always been happy to discuss it.

CHAPTER 5

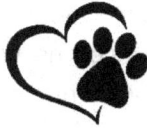

Common Issues Support

WHEN YOU ARE THE GUARDIAN OF AN ANIMAL, you will have
issues that come up that you need to address for the optimum
health of your animal. Most people think you must be in person to
give and receive a healing session, but healing works whether you
are in the same room together or not.

Remote Healing

Everything is energy. In physics, we learn that energy does not
know time or space. That means I can be anywhere and work with
a client in another city, state, or country as if we are in the same
room. This is how I am able to support feral cats, fearful animals,
aggressive animals, and animals that do not like to be touched, and
get the same results as if I could touch them.

Animals know what they want and when they want it.

Early on in my career, I had a regular dog client, Cerne. He would
receive weekly, in-person healing sessions. I went on vacation to
Cancun, Mexico. I was awoken at 5:30 a.m., feeling an energy

hovering over my bed to get my attention. I was quite surprised and curious. Never having encountered this before and being half asleep, I was figuring out how to handle this situation. I rubbed my eyes to make sure I was seeing what I was seeing. Cerne was energetically hovering over the bed. I recognized his energy and saw a visual of him. I noticed he was pointing to his right hip, communicating that it was hurting, and he wanted healing support. And he wanted it at that moment. My first thought was, *I am on vacation, how did he find me?* And the next thought was, *it is 5:30 a.m., and I was sleeping; couldn't we do it when I was awake?*

I decided to help him. I sat up, connected with him, and supported his right hip. He was very happy and merrily went on his way, and I went back to sleep. I was still processing the reality of what had just transpired. I had heard remote sessions were possible, but now I knew for sure. This opened the door for me to offer remote healing sessions to clients wherever they live.

Another time this happened was with a regular cat client, Satchit. This time, it was not a foreign concept to me. He was home alone in New York City (with a pet sitter checking in and taking care of him) while his guardians were away visiting family. It was Thanksgiving Day. He came to me scared and freaked out. I stepped away from my family visit to help him. I connected, communicated with him, did calming techniques, and got him settled and calm. He was content and happy.

And another time, I was interrupted in the shower by regular cat client, Moonbeam, from Santa Fe, New Mexico. She wanted her energetic protection support reinforced. She had been receiving that support in her private healing sessions and liked it. I laughed that I had no privacy in the shower. The shower is where I set my energy for the day, and after I set my protections (as you learned in Chapter 2), I supported Moonbeam. She was grateful and went on about her business. I did too.

Energy is energy. That is the language of animals. What I have found is that animals I work with during remote healing sessions know me when I meet them in person (just as I knew Cerne when he visited me in Mexico). I had the privilege of meeting some of my regular remote clients, Satchit in New York City, Mickey and Moonbeam in Santa Fe, Levi in Olathe, Kansas, and Kiya in Seattle.

I had been supporting cat client, Kiya, with distance-healing wellness sessions. When I attended a party at her guardian's house, Kiya recognized me. I had my food in one hand, water in the other, and she kept nudging my hands with her head profusely. So, I put the food and water down, Kiya sat in my lap, curled up in my hands, and was happily soaking in the healing energy.

Animals know what they need, when they need it, and ask for it. They do not stop themselves from asking. As people, we can learn a lot from animals in this way.

Calming, Feeling Safe, and Building Trust

For your cat and dog, it is important for them to have a safe spot they can go when they are feeling scared or unsure.

Here are two healing techniques powerful on their own and are highly beneficial when used together.

Grounding Hold on Sacrum (Low Back)

This is especially great for fearful animals.

Lightly place your whole hand on the low back of your animal. This light touch that is stationary is called the passive touch massage stroke, which is the only massage stroke that is safe to do across the spine. You will have part of your hand on top of one hip, one part of your hand across the low back, and one part of your hand on top of the other hip. This is an extra gentle placement of your hand resting lightly on your animal's low back.

This is exceptionally grounding and provides a gentle calming. This is especially good to support fearful animals to feel safer and begin to relax.

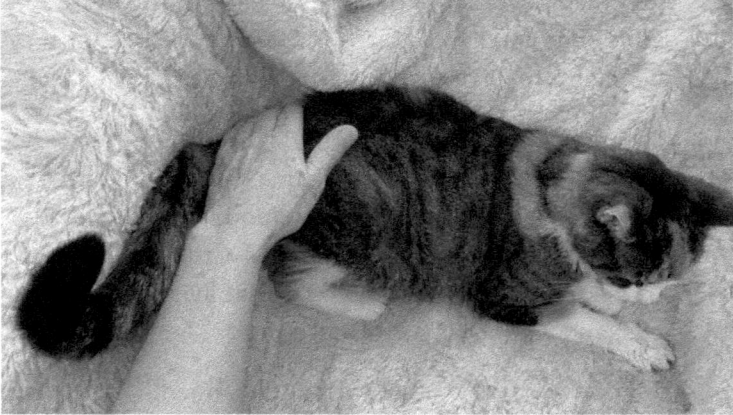

Grounding Sacrum Hold

To enhance the grounding and calming for your pet, use your other hand to hold the CV17—Center of chest.

CV17—Center of chest

The acupressure point CV17 stands for Central Vessel 17, also called Conception Vessel 17, and is located in the center of the chest.

Place your whole hand on the center of your animal's chest. You are engaging the CV17 acupressure point, along with your hand connecting to the heart chakra. This is the passive touch massage stroke when you place your hand on the body gently and hold. It is calming to your animal for your hand to be placed on his/her chest.

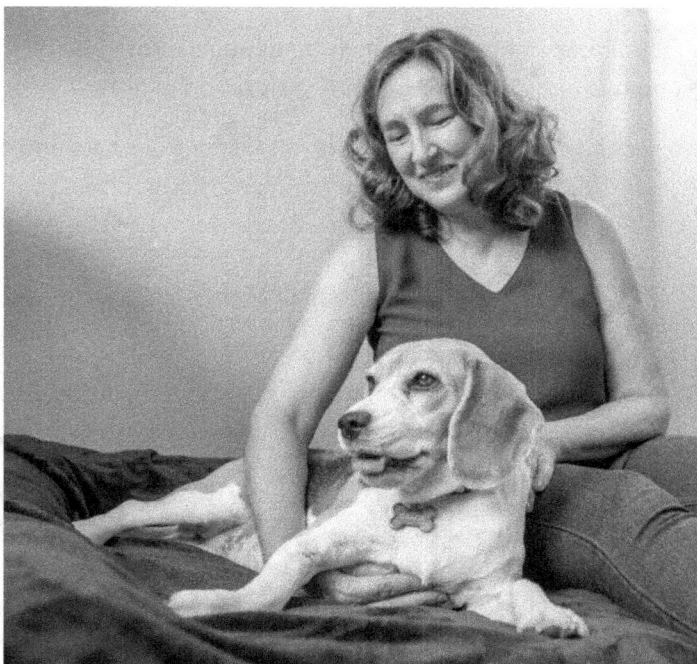

Holding the Heart CV17 Point

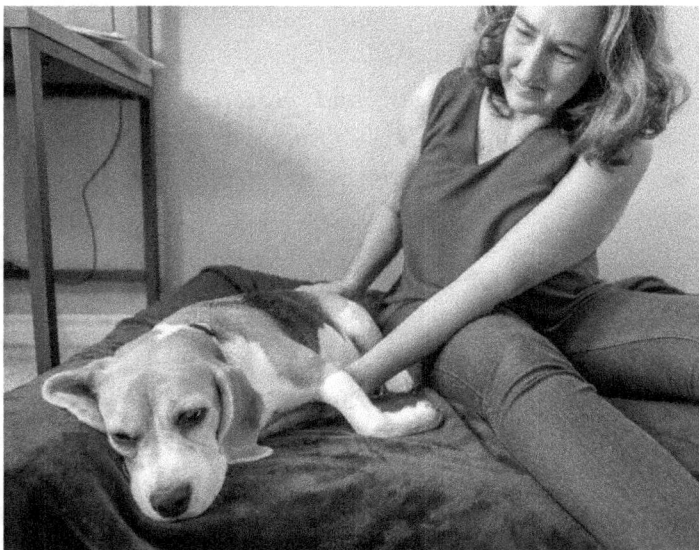

Holding the Heart CV17 Point and Sacrum at the Same Time

Common Issues, Especially With Rescue Animals

The techniques in this section can be beneficial for your cats and dogs, no matter what their beginning situation in life has been.

These techniques are especially important for your cats and dogs who have come from a shelter or foster environment, been rehomed, or who have had multiple homes in their life.

Rescue Cats Generally Come With Colds

Kittens and cats coming from shelters will most likely have a cold. It is a fact. Clear drainage is generally not a concern. If the eyes get goopy, or nasal discharge has a color, you will need to see a veterinarian.

In Spirit's and Sapphire's case, they received their adoption wellness veterinarian examination, and the sneezing and clear drainage lasted more than a couple of weeks. They took a lysine supplement with their food to help boost their immune systems.

❧ *Your Essence Experience* ❧

For extra support with Spirit and Sapphire, I used the Healing Your Animal **Clear, Iceland Spar,** *and* **Protection** *essences. These provide a simple, effective, easy-to-use way to calm and balance you and your pet while boosting health. Simply spray the essence three times in the air around you and your pet two to three times a day.*

When researching Lysine supplements, only get pure lysine. The gels and supplements that the veterinarians and even animal health food stores carry contain ingredients to avoid, such as artificial sweeteners and soy. Especially in the case of having young kittens with compromised immune systems, my goal was to help strengthen their systems. I was so surprised and disappointed to discover the unhealthy ingredients.

At the time, NOW brand carried a pure lysine supplement for humans, and Thorne brand had a lysine with leucine supplement for humans that was made from good ingredients to give your kittens and cats. (I cleared this with my holistic veterinarian). Please read the ingredients, as things may have changed since the writing of this book. And always when starting a new supplement, please get the advice and dosage from your veterinarian.

Note: If you are using a supplement made for humans to administer to your pets, you must get the proper dosing from your veterinarian. In general, you will use much less for your pet than for yourself.

I have found it is easier to start with lower dosages than recommended, mixing the powder into the pet food and then building up to the recommended dosage. The reason is that lysine has a bitter taste, and you want your animals to eat the food with the supplement.

Sapphire and Spirit readily ate their food with the lysine, so I was grateful. And their sneezing and drainage stopped.

They had even more kitten energy to rumble, tumble, and get into mischief.

Helping Your Pet Stay Calm in Life Situations

One of the things you need to be aware of when you have adopted a rescue animal is that they are really on edge because of an unstable home environment.

Things such as these can easily upset them:

- Going to the veterinarian
- Going to the groomer
- When you leave the house, and they are left behind
- People coming over to your house

- Having a cat sitter

- Having a dog sitter

- Going to doggie day care

- Taking a trip to the park

- Them leaving with a pet walker

- Visiting other people's homes with your pet

These activities are all overly stressful to your rescued pet, especially those that have had multiple residences before you.

Since they have been rehomed, they do not know what is happening. They may get anxious because they do not know that when you leave the house, you are coming back. They do not know when you leave them at the vet, groomer's, and doggie day care, you are coming back to pick them up. They do not know they are coming back home with you when you visit a friend's house or a park together. They do not know if someone else is going to take them home or take them somewhere else as others have done in the past.

The good news is that there is a way to communicate your intentions to them.

One of the simplest ways to communicate with your pet is to visualize a scenario. Show them a picture in your mind of what you desire them to see.

In these scenarios, make sure you "show and tell" them you are going together and coming home together. And when your friend is visiting, tell your pet that your friend will go home, and the two of you are staying in your forever home together.

Animals do not know what day and night means. Day to them is light outside. Night is dark outside. To communicate the number of days and nights that you will be gone, show them with blinks of your eyes. One blink equals one night.

Making Veterinarian Trips

Veterinarian trips can cause stress for both you and your pet.

It is important to "show and tell" your pet that you are going to the veterinarian and coming back home together.

A special note for cat guardians:

Take both cats to the veterinarian, even if the doctor will see only one cat.

Smells your cat brings home from the veterinarian can trigger another cat that stayed home to not recognize him or her after coming home. This can lead to fights and cause a lot of stress in the household.

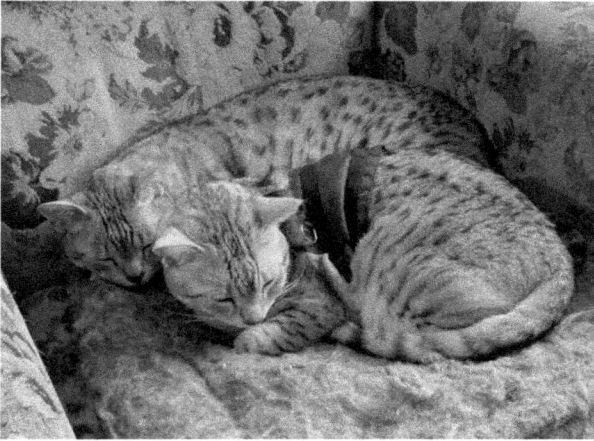

Anubis and Ramses

In some instances, it may take cats a few days to get along again. Others may take longer. Anubis and Ramses took two and a half years to start to cuddle and three and a half years to snuggle comfortably again.

If your pet must stay overnight at the veterinarian, communicate this with your pet, showing blinks for how long and reassuring your pet that he/she will be coming back home to you (only if this is true).

For example, your pet is going to be at the veterinarian for one night and coming home the next day during daylight hours. You show your pet one blink, and then show them in your mind that you are picking them up and going home together.

The passive touch technique discussed in the beginning of this chapter can be used anytime when your pet is stressed—for example, on the way to the veterinarian, feeling ill, a new environment. Placing your hand on your pet's chest and/or low back is recommended. If you are unable to get to either of those areas, calmly and gently place your hand where your pet is comfortable being touched. Be sure to place both hands on your pet for a two-handed connection and extra calming.

❧ *Your Essence Experience* ❧

*For extra support, the Healing Your Animal **Serene** essence is a natural, effective, easy-to-use way to calm you and your pet. Simply spray the essence three times in the air around you and your pet before you leave the house, when you get in the car, and when you get to the veterinarian clinic to receive calming support. (My clients that have asked to spray the essences during their veterinarian visits have been welcomed to use the essences.)*

❧ *Your Essence Experience* ❧

*For extra support, the Healing Your Animal **Iceland Spar** essence is a natural, effective, easy-to-use way to calm and balance you and your pet. This has been effective in reducing car sickness for pets. Simply spray the essence three times in the air around you and your pet before you leave the house, when you get in the car, and when you get to the veterinarian clinic to receive calming and balancing support. (My clients that have asked to spray the essences during their veterinarian visits have been welcomed to use the essences.)*

Traveling Away From Your Pet

Cats Vincent and Pablo have been long-time clients. Sally and her husband, their guardians, travel frequently, and some trips are longer than others are. For the big trips especially, Sally wants to ensure that Vincent and Pablo understand the plans, knowing they will relax and do better while she is away. It is especially helpful when there is a new pet sitter taking care of them. Sally has sitters come meet the cats before she leaves. And when I share with the cats who will be taking care of them, they relax. They like to know who will be coming to feed them and play with them. Sally makes sure she and the cats like the sitters before she leaves.

It is important to be mindful about having someone care for your pet(s) while you travel. There are times animals have shown me it was not the best situation for them. And on some level, the guardian has known this to be true, but ignored their intuition. Find a reputable and bonded pet sitter, introduce your pets to them before you leave, and communicate your travel plans to make your travel for both your pets and you more relaxing.

As I explained before, to communicate the number of days and nights you will be away from your pet, you show them with blinks of your eyes.

For example, you are going away for three nights and coming back on the fourth day during the daytime, and you are leaving in five days, so that is four nights together before you leave:

- Visualize yourself and your pet together for four more nights, then show them four blinks.

- Visualize yourself leaving out the door with your suitcase.

- Show your pet three blinks.

- Then visualize yourself coming back home, walking through the door with your suitcase.

Tip: I recommend you giving pets a heads up about your travel plans. They are sensitive and know you are doing something. They just do not know what yet. It would be nice to tell them before you bring out your suitcase.

I have some clients, such as Sally with cats Vincent and Pablo, who, after being taught the communicating travel technique, still prefer for me to communicate the travel plans with their pet(s) to ensure a good trip. This relieves any worry on the guardian's part about their pets receiving the message of their guardian's trip details clearly. The pets appreciate knowing they are being taken care of, who is taking care of them while their guardian is away, and knowing when their guardian is coming home. This goes for when you are traveling with your pet too.

Traveling With Your Pet

As you are preparing for your trip with your pet, it is important to let them know what is happening so they will be more relaxed.

To communicate the number of days and nights that you will be away together with your pet, show them with the blinks of your eyes.

For example, say you are traveling for three nights and coming back on the fourth day during the daytime. You are leaving in five days, so that is four nights in your home together before you leave:

- To show your pet that you are together for four more nights in your home, visualize you and your pet together, and show them four blinks.
- Then picture the both of you leaving out the door with your suitcase, getting in the (airplane, train, etc.).
- Show your pet three blinks to indicate the time you will be gone.
- Picture you and your pet coming back home together, through the door of your home with your suitcase.

Tip: I recommend you giving your pet a heads up about your travel plans even when it includes them. They are sensitive and know you are doing something, but they just do not know what yet. And they do not know they are included. It would be nice to tell them before you bring out your suitcase.

Lifestyle Changes

Moving with Your Pet

When you are getting ready to move, you know you have a new home. You know you must box up everything and transport it to your new home. You have a big to-do list. However, your animals do not know what is happening. Their world is being turned upside down. While you know your animal is going with you to your new home, your pet does not. You need to specifically tell them.

I brought Tasha home from the pound when she was seven weeks old. She had moved across the country with me from Huntsville, Alabama, to Kirkland, Washington. She moved to California with me when I moved to the Bay Area. She moved back to Seattle with me when my husband Peter and I decided to come back to Seattle to raise a family. In this time, she lived in hotels and temporary housing with us until we found a home. When I got divorced, she moved out to an apartment with me. When I bought a house, she moved with me.

When I was moving to another house, I was boxing up things, and Tasha was acting funny. I could not figure it out, and I was concerned. I called the animal communicator that I use for my animals when it is hard to fully read my own situation, being so close to it. She told me Tasha did not know she was moving with me. I said, "What? Of course, she is coming with me!" When I specifically told her, she calmed down, and the move went smoothly. On this move, I took it for granted that she knew she was coming with me. I learned how important it is to tell animals everything that is impacting their world. Once they understand, they relax.

When One Pet Dies While Another Pet Is Still Alive

When one pet passes, it is easy to be consumed with the grief, and the other pet does not understand.

Two pugs, Lucy and Linus, grew up together. Lucy was the alpha, and Linus depended on Lucy for security. Lucy got sick and later died. This left Linus scared, skittish, and having separation anxiety. In their grief, Linus' guardians were feeling bad for Linus not having Lucy around. Linus did not understand why they were feeling bad toward him. (From his world, they were looking at him and being concerned, worried, and sad. He was confused as to why). I communicated with Linus about the grief his guardians were feeling. When he realized that he was okay, and he was not doing anything wrong, he could relax.

Linus' guardians were extra conscientious. They were worried about leaving Linus alone at home, knowing he was having trouble with separation anxiety. I educated them to not be worried when leaving. If they were worried, that gave Linus a reason to worry. They shifted to being more confident, leaving Linus at home while they ran errands. Leaving a worn, unwashed piece of clothing with their scent on it helped Linus to feel safer. I communicated with Linus that his guardians are coming back when they leave, and he relaxed.

Another shift that needed to happen with his guardians and their grief that was important to Linus was being greeted in the morning. Linus slept with his guardians. When they got up in the morning, they would say "hi" to Lucy in her urn, but not to Linus. They knew Linus was there, so did not think anything about it. Once they started greeting Linus too, he was more content.

It is a balancing act, managing your grief over the loss of your beloved pet, and sharing joy and love with your pet who is still alive.

Common Health Issues

Allergies

Allergies can be caused by multiple sources.

Food (the list is extensive), indoor environment such as dust, dirt, mold, mildew, and outside items such as grass, trees, pollen, and more.

With cat client, Sin, I discovered that not all raw foods are created equal. Sin had patches of fur missing on parts of her body. She would scratch a lot. With her healing sessions, she had cleared and balanced her body, which reduced her itching; yet it was still hanging on. We dove deeper into talking about her food and narrowed down what source of proteins her body would easily digest and accept. She was already eating raw (which can result in a significant jump in health benefits). Honoring the specific proteins her body would easily accept helped some. Yet again, Sin was not fully having the itching go away. So, I had Sin's guardian switch raw food brands to Natural Pet Pantry. They are strict about the quality of ingredients that go into their food. It worked! Sin got better. It turns out that Sin was reacting to a synthetic ingredient the other company had added to their food.

- **LI11 Acupressure Point**

  Acupressure point LI11 is used to relieve allergies. Lift the foot, flex the elbow, and find the crease that forms on the outside of the elbow. Feel for the depression at the end of the crease, just in front of the bony prominence.

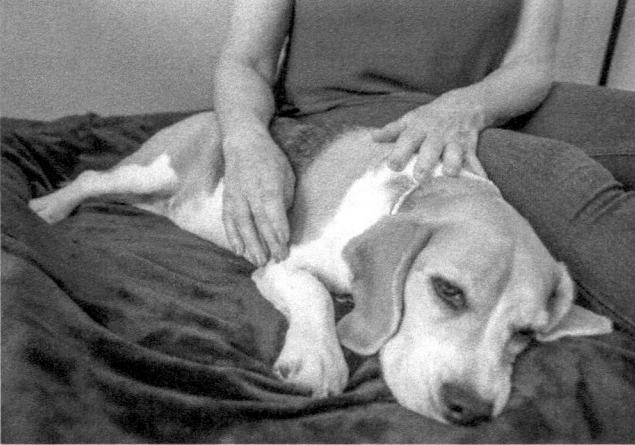

Holding the LI11 Point

Digestive Issues

It is important to have good gut health for your animal. Sometimes adding probiotics or goat's milk to your pet's diet will support healthy digestion. Always get the proper dosing from your veterinarian.

❧ *Your Essence Experience* ❧

For extra support, use the Healing Your Animal **Digestion Ease** *essence for an effective, easy-to-use way to support healthy digestion. Simply spray the essence three times in the air around your pet two to three times a day at mealtime.*

See sections below for natural support for constipation and diarrhea specifically.

Constipation

If constipation starts, here are some natural techniques to help get bowels moving. Contact your veterinarian for monitoring instructions. You want to be sure that your pet does not have a blockage and know-how to determine when you need to take them into the veterinarian for support.

The first thing to try is to add water to your pet's food.

The second thing to try is one tablespoon of canned pumpkin to add fiber to your pet's diet. (With finicky animals, start with a smaller amount. For my cats, I started with a quarter teaspoon so they would eat it.)

Acupressure Points to Stimulate

See Acupressure in the Definitions section at the beginning of the book for instructions.

- **LI4 Acupressure Point**

    Acupressure point LI4 is located inside the first toe, in the web between the dewclaw or where the dewclaw would be. LI4 balances the gastrointestinal system.

    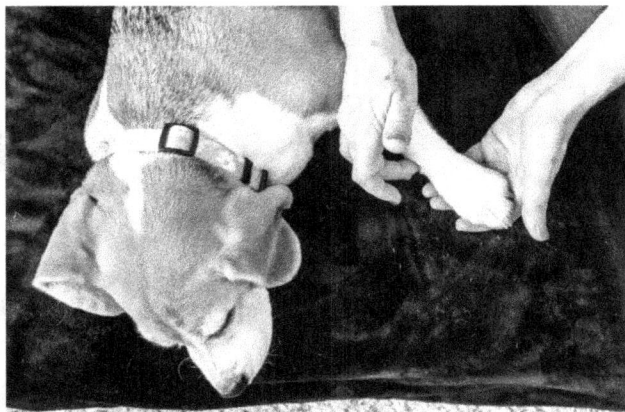

    Holding the LI4 Point

- **SP6 Acupressure Point**

    Acupressure point SP6 is located on the inside of the lower back leg, three cun above the tip of the ankle bone, on the back of the shin bone. SP6 is the Master point for the lower abdomen.

Vicki Draper

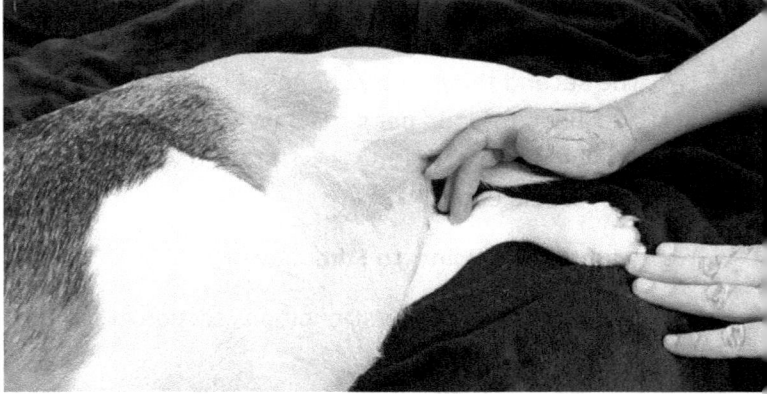

Holding the SP6 Point

- **ST36 Acupressure Point**

  Acupressure point ST36 is located on the outside hind leg, just below the knee, in a depression in the middle of the muscle toward the front of the leg. ST36 is the Master Point for the abdomen and gastrointestinal tract.

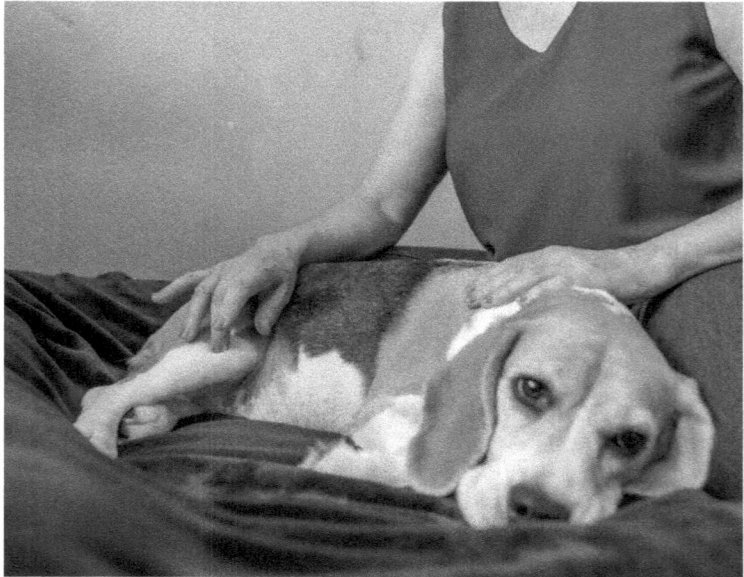

Holding the ST36 Point

Diarrhea

If diarrhea starts, talk to your veterinarian to get monitoring instructions. You want to prevent dehydration in your pet.

Here are some natural techniques to use in the meantime.

- **LI4 Acupressure Point**

  Acupressure point LI4 is located inside the first toe, in the web between the dewclaw or where the dewclaw would be. LI4 balances the gastrointestinal system.

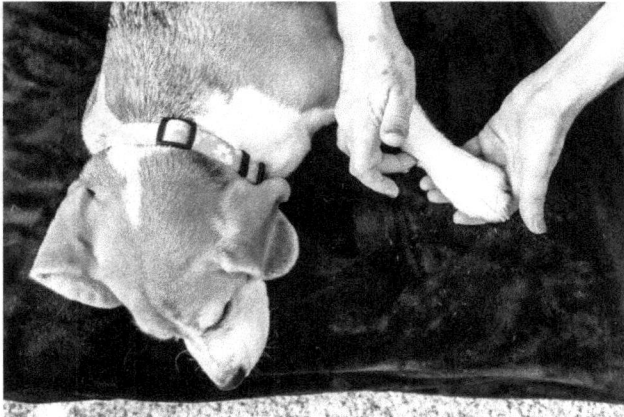

Holding the LI 4 Point

- **SP6 Acupressure Point**

  Acupressure point SP6 is located on the inside of the lower back leg, three cun above the tip of the ankle bone, on the back of the shin bone. SP6 is the Master point for the lower abdomen.

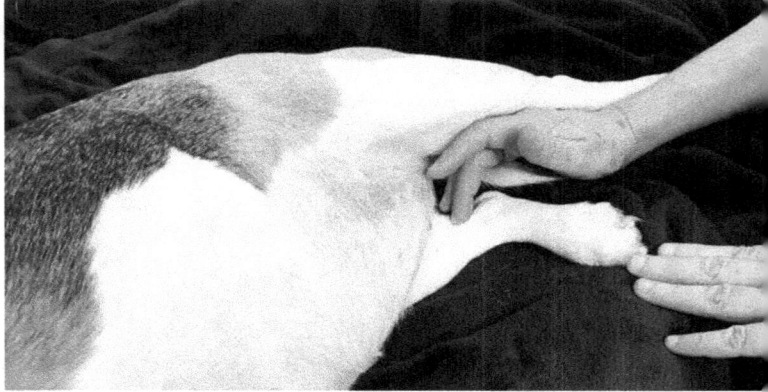

Holding the SP6 Point

- **ST25 Acupressure Point**

  Use ST25 for gastrointestinal disorders and to relieve diarrhea. It is located on each side of the belly button. For cats and small dogs, use one finger width. For medium-size dogs, use two finger widths. For large dogs, use three finger widths. Typically, cat and dog belly buttons appear as flat scars without hair, located in the middle of the abdomen, midway between the abdomen and the hips.

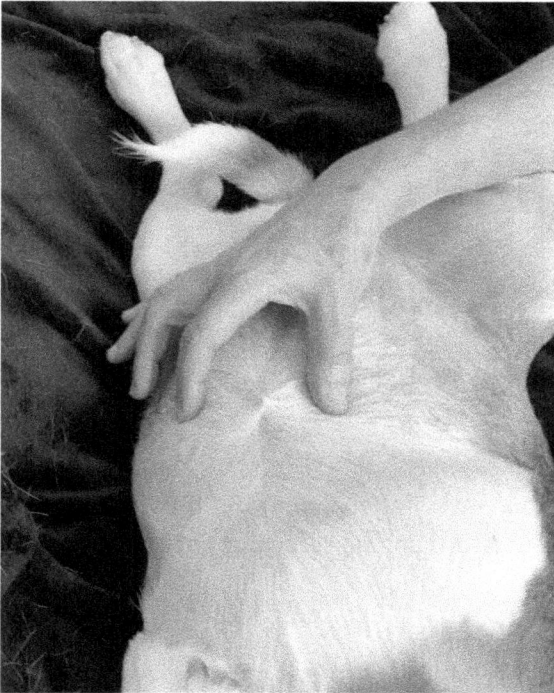

Holding the ST25Point

- **ST36 Acupressure Point**

  Acupressure point ST36 is located on the outside hind leg, just below the knee, in a depression in the middle of the muscle toward the front of the leg. ST36 is the Master Point for the abdomen and gastrointestinal tract.

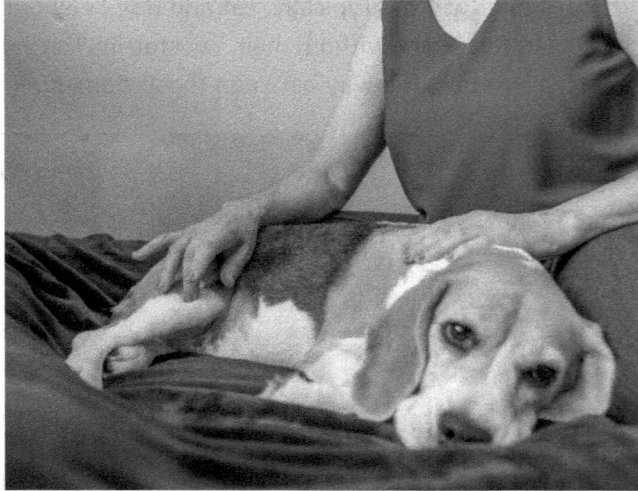

Holding the ST36 Point

Vomiting

Talk to your veterinarian if your pet is vomiting. You want to rule out serious issues and be sure your pet does not get dehydrated.

Once those issues are ruled out, the source of the problem could be stress or food.

As you may remember from Chapter 2, my cat Tasha was throwing up, and the veterinarian confirmed there was not anything physically wrong with her. I then discovered she was reacting to my stress.

Vomiting can also be a reaction to food. I had a cat client, Olivia, who had been throwing up regularly. Energy testing the food she was eating showed it was not a good protein source for her to digest easily. After she changed protein sources, she was keeping her food down and feeling much better. Sometimes it can be an ingredient in the food. The fewer ingredients in the food the better for your pet's digestion, especially when they are having sensitivities already.

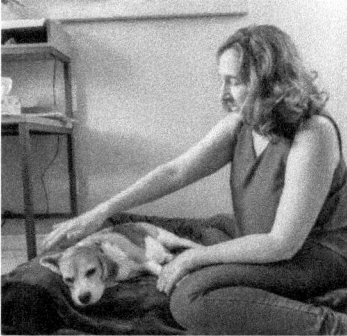

Step 1

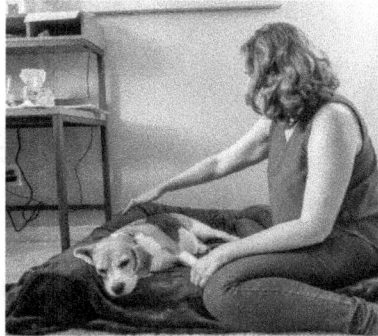

Step 2

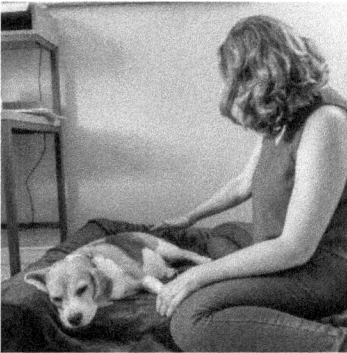

Step 3

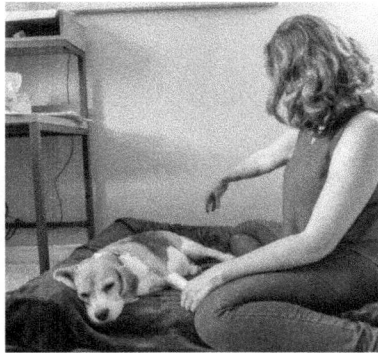

Step 4

Tip to Tail Technique

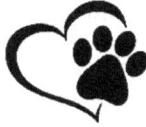

CHAPTER 6

Serious Health Issues

ONE OF THE BENEFITS of having a regular grounding and centering routine is it helps you get clearer more quickly in times of crisis and emergency.

This is why I recommend you have a daily grounding practice. When there is a crisis, you can manage it more calmly and clearly.

The following sections detail how you can support yourself and your pet through specific health situations.

Amputation

There are circumstances when your pet needs to go through amputation. Many emotions that come up when your animal goes through amputation. Your animal notices and responds to your emotions.

A dog client, Toby, had cancer, and had to have one leg amputated. What struck me then is what a wonderful, cheerful personality he had. He actually had a smile on his face, even after what he had just been through. My initial session with him was focused on not only the physical healing that was happening but his energy as well. There was a huge flood of his guardian's worry and emotions coming through his amputation area that were releasing while I was working on his newly amputated leg. I was not prepared for that. The energy was so strong that I was almost pushed over by it.

Our animals are sensitive to our energies and do not always understand them. In that initial session, Toby asked me what he had done wrong. He could not understand why his guardians were looking at him hurting, sad, and worried.

Once we cleared and balanced this for him, it gave him clarity, and he perked up and was much happier. It also shifted the energy of the guardians. They could look at Toby in a much stronger light than they had before.

It was great to watch this loving bond go to an even deeper level between them. The session brought an even closer connection and understanding between them. By the time Toby left his session, he had a bigger smile on his face.

Toby came for routine sessions. He continued to have his smile and upbeat disposition. Toby is such a clear example of how to take life in stride, stay calm and happy during our adversities.

Maggie, a pointer, was an agility dog who had cancer in her leg, so it had to be amputated. The amputation ended her agility career. Her guardian was ashamed and disappointed. I shared with her guardian that Maggie was still a full dog. She would learn to walk on three legs and still be her loving self. Her guardian was in such grief that the information was not registering. She was not seeing Maggie as being a wonderful, complete dog.

Animals are aware of their guardians' emotions. Our pets are like sponges with our emotions, and we are not aware of it. Seeing their guardians upset, both Toby and Maggie wanted to know what they did wrong. I educated them that they had done nothing wrong.

❧ *Your Essence Experience* ❧

*For extra support, use the Healing Your Animal **Pain Ease** essence. It is a natural, effective, easy-to-use way to support easing your emotional pain when your pet is going through something serious like amputation. It is a soothing balm, helping nurture your emotional pain. Simply spray the essence three times in the surrounding air to receive emotional pain support.*

❧ *Your Essence Experience* ❧

*For extra support, use Healing Your Animal **Protection** essence, a natural, effective, easy-to-use way to protect your animal from your emotions when your animal is going through a serious issue. Simply spray the essence three times in the air around your animal to benefit from protection support.*

Paralysis

Kathy and Brent first started working with me when Samson, their eight-year-old cocker spaniel, fell off the bed one morning. Samson was paralyzed and could not walk. She had taken Samson to the veterinarian, and he had also received acupuncture with no noticeable improvement. Kathy and Brent had to hold Samson up to go potty, as he could not stand on his own.

Kathy was unfamiliar with distance-healing sessions; yet, she was desperate, so she started working with me. After Samson's first session, I instructed her to take him out to potty, as the session would be processing through him, and he would need to pee. Within five minutes after his first session, Kathy and Brent took Samson out to go potty. He was able to stand and pee on his own! Their jaws dropped open from sheer amazement. This was such great relief for Kathy and Brent. We worked more together, and Samson continued to full recovery, walking and running again.

Ingesting a Toxic Substance

Sally's cats, Vincent and Pablo, both got into something toxic. The experience at the veterinarian was extremely unsettling, especially for Pablo. He scrambled up and broke the blinds. Sally decided to see if I could help them since going to the veterinarian had been so traumatic for Vincent and Pablo. Sally and I stayed in close communication, and the cats responded to their healing sessions. They kept improving. They were able to heal without the additional emergency veterinarian trip. Sally, Vincent, and Pablo were all relieved for this support.

I recommend that you see your veterinarian when your animal gets into something toxic.

Acupressure Detox

Here is a detox method in support of veterinarian care for ingesting toxic substances and for mild issues such as changing food.

- **LI4, LV3 Acupressure Points**

   On the diagonal of the body, use LI4 on the front left paw and LV3 on the back right paw simultaneously, then switch to LI4 on the front right paw and LV3 on the back left paw simultaneously.

   Acupressure point LI4 is located inside the first toe, in the web between the dewclaw or where the dewclaw would be.

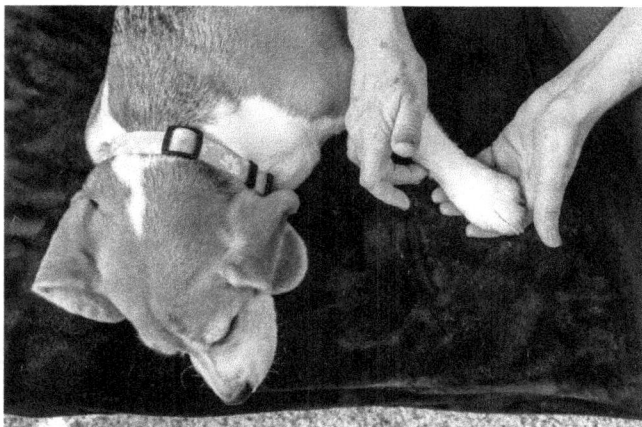

Holding the LI4 Point

Acupressure point Lv3 is located on the top of the back paw in the webbing between the first and second toes.

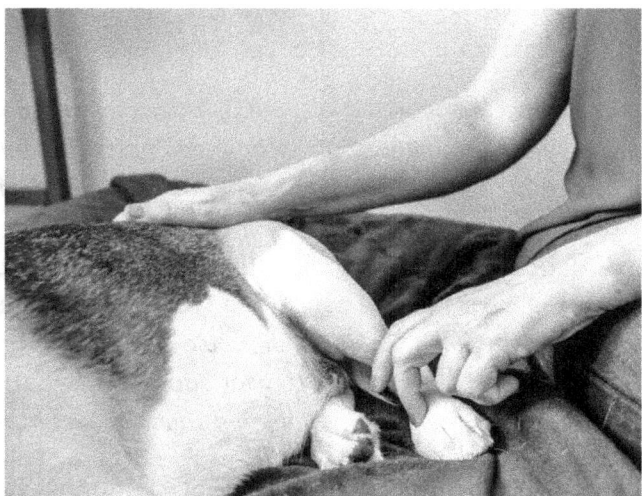

Holding the LV3 Point

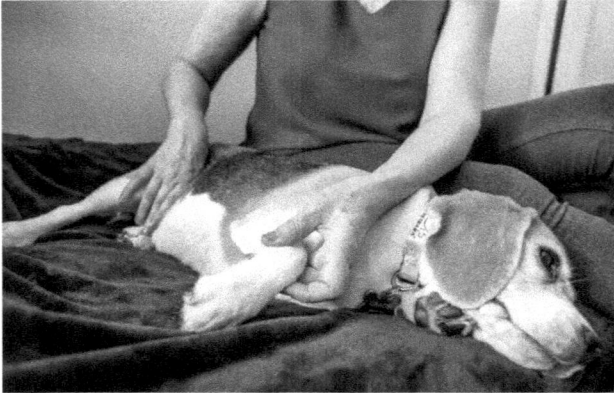

Holding the LI4 with LV3 Points on Opposite Sides

Cat Surviving a Dog Attack

Not all cats survive being attacked by a dog. Here is one cat that did.

Client April shares the story of her cat, Ali:

"I have really valued working with Vicki, especially since my cat Ali was attacked by a neighbor's dog and was not expected to live. Ali's jaw was broken (the dog had her head in his mouth and shook her violently before I interrupted the attack). After dealing with animal control and requesting spiritual support through prayer, I texted Vicki as I was on the way to the vet. The initial impression from the veterinarian was that Ali would not survive (and they were shocked she didn't have internal damage when the X-rays came back). Then the veterinarian said that she would probably not be able to feed herself after they watched her for 24 hours, and thought they would need to wire her jaw shut and put her on a feeding tube.

After 24 hours (she was in shock and being given fluids by the animal hospital), the staff were stunned that Ali was able to eat on her own, and they stated she was lapping the food up like a dog! I took her home and had two sessions with Vicki where she helped first with the shock and trauma, and then with physical issues that resulted from the incident. Vicki was able to tune in energetically to the physical issues even though I hadn't specified yet that Ali was compensating in her walking due to muscle injury.

Two weeks after the incident, my cat was back to her old self, with a permanently misaligned jaw, but not needing the extensive dental surgeries that her surgeon thought she might need. She is an old cat, 15 years, and now she lives indoors, but she is happy and healthy, and adjusted beautifully after spending most of her life with the freedom of the outdoors. I am grateful I had Vicki as a resource through this experience, and the veterinarian staff were amazed at the rapid recovery of Ali, especially given her age. Today Ali spends her days sleeping on my lap as I work from home or antagonizing her brother (a seven-year-old Bichon). Thank you, Vicki!"

—April Choulat

Loss of Appetite

It is time to get concerned when your animal stops eating. This is the time to see your veterinarian immediately.

Cats especially need to get veterinarian attention immediately because cats hide their health issues, and it could be something serious.

A technique to use in addition to veterinarian care is:

- **ST36 Acupressure Point**

  Acupressure point ST36 is located on the outside hind leg, just below the knee, in a depression in the middle of the muscle toward the front of the leg. ST36 is the Master Point for the abdomen and gastrointestinal tract.

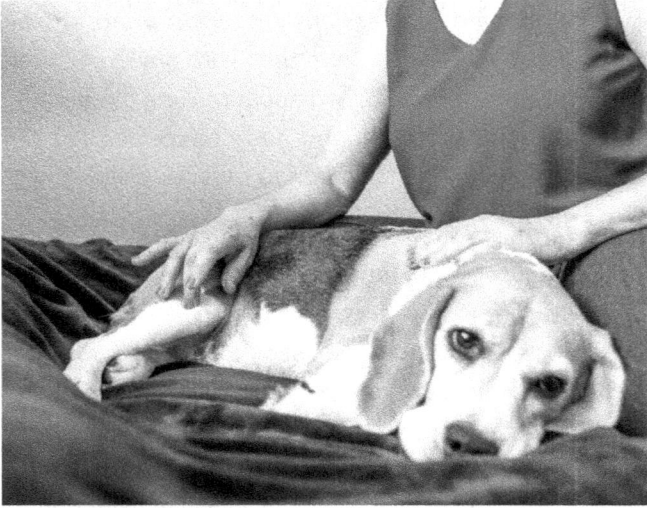

Holding the ST36 Point

Massage Ears

Stimulate your pet's ears by gently massaging them. See if this increases interest and ability to eat more food.

Boost Appetite

Anyone who has gone through a loss of appetite with a pet has experienced picky eating. You may have found yourself offering many different foods to see what your pet will eat. One day your pet likes a food, and the next day they do not. You are not alone.

Make sure your pet has enough water, since your animal can sustain health, feel better, and live longer while hydrated.

Here are some things to help boost your animal's appetite naturally to see if you can get more food into your pet.

Smelly food

Your pet will generally go for smellier foods such as tripe, tuna, sardines, and liver treats.

Fresh food

Shannon's beagle dog client, Scooby, liked food that was right out of the oven, a dog food recipe called meatloaf, consisting of meat, veggies, and digestive enzymes made especially for him.

- **ST36 Acupressure Point**

  Acupressure point ST36 is located on the outside hind leg, just below the knee, in a depression in the middle of the muscle toward the front of the leg. ST36 is the Master Point for the abdomen and gastrointestinal tract.

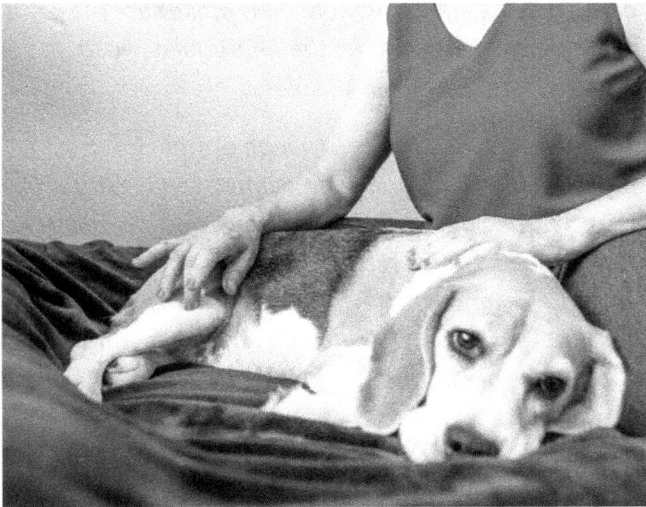

Holding the ST36 Point

❧ Your Essence Experience ❧

*For extra support, the Healing Your Animal **Appetite** essence is a natural, effective, easy-to-use way to support increasing your animal's appetite. Simply spray the essence three times in the air around your animal and their food to receive boosting appetite support.*

Kidney Issues

Cats are more notorious for having kidney issues; however, it can also happen in dogs.

Wisdom from my interview with Nancy Howard, Owner of Whole Cat & Kaboodle and Founder and Director of Feral Care Sanctuary:

"There is a prevailing myth that cats with kidney issues need less protein. But that is not true. Yes, kidneys can be damaged by the metabolic waste from protein, so what we do not want to do is to limit the amount of protein because these animals are obligate carnivores. What we want to do is make sure the cat is eating clean protein, so we manage the metabolic waste through a clean protein instead of a dirty protein.

"What is a clean protein? A clean protein is a fresh, not denatured protein, raw food, and even canned food. With raw food, there is anecdotal evidence that it can buy back kidney function. But we know that in dry foods, the proteins are filthy because they are denatured, and many of those proteins are coming from grain products instead of meat products. And no matter what anyone says, those are different amino acid profiles you cannot get around that."

Serious Illness and Cancer

Sophie, a five-year-old miniature poodle, had serious health issues, yet maintained a fun, perky disposition. She was cute, spunky, and had a diva attitude. She was so smart, and she loved her healing sessions.

Sophie was getting a lot of attention from her guardian and receiving many healing sessions due to recovering from cancer, diabetes, pancreatitis, thrombocytopenia, and vasculitis. She had metastatic mammary gland carcinoma, aka breast cancer, which spread locally three times, involving the vascular and lymph system.

In one session, she showed me having fun, flying like an angel in a yellow cape with a red S. She wanted to help animals with hope, as she had been through a lot in her life. I asked if she wanted to be part of my book so she could help more animals. She gave me a resounding yes.

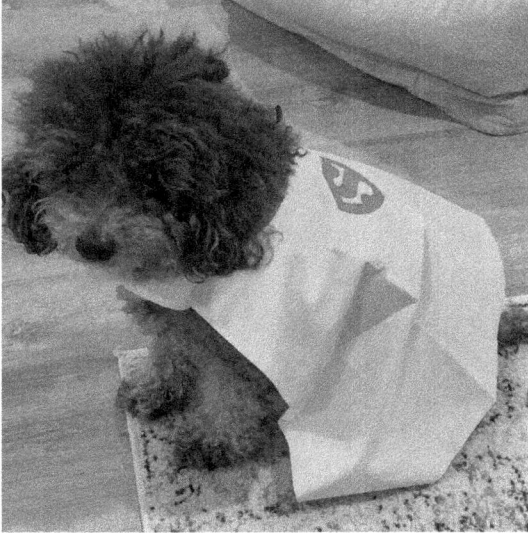

Sophie—photo submitted by Claire Jai

Sophie directed her sessions, telling me where to work, when to work, and for how long.

At the end of her sessions, I always asked her if there were any other areas that she needed support with before we ended her session. Usually there was a spot she wanted to be addressed, so I would focus on that then end her session.

One day, when I asked her this question, she showed me a spot in her lower pelvic region.

When I started working there, she was not ready to allow it to clear. She said she did not want to leave.

She figured out my pattern and wanted to hang out longer for her session. I thought that was so sweet. I told her she would be coming back for more sessions, so she happily released and balanced.

In one session, Sophie shared that she was afraid of getting better; that she would lose the closely monitored attention she was getting from her guardian. Her guardian and I assured Sophie that she could continue her healing sessions and receive lots of attention from her guardian when she was healthier, so she could let herself heal.

This is actually very common. You have a routine and pattern together with your pet, and your pet wants to be sure you really want it to change. Your pet looks to you to get permission to heal, and then chooses to allow the healing to take place.

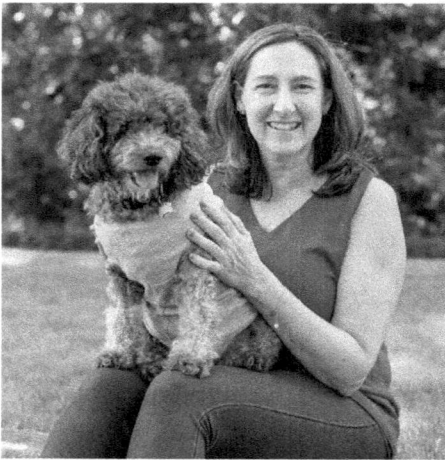

Sophie with Vicki the day after cancer surgery

When cancer diagnosis, I advise you to consult with your veterinarian before doing the Healing Session Protocol (described in Chapter 3).

Passive touch, Reiki, and clearing techniques do not involve manual manipulation, and generally are safe to use when cancer is involved.

Cancer Support

When working with Susan's kitten, I found an issue with her. I suggested she go to the veterinarian. When she did go to the veterinarian, her kitten had cancer.

Cancer. When you get the diagnosis, your heart may sink; you may see your animal's life passing before your eyes, thinking it is all over with your pet.

There is good news, though. Animals can recover from some cancers. There are many factors to consider: some types of cancer are more aggressive than others, some are systemic, and some are local.

When getting this diagnosis, it can be a tough decision about whether to do chemotherapy and/or radiation or not.

Something to keep in mind is that animals do not think the way we do. There is no wrong answer to them. Yes, they love you and want to be with you. They are not afraid of death (I also call this transitioning). They accept it as a natural part of life.

It comes down to personal preference of how you desire to treat the cancer.

Some things to consider are:

- The age and stamina of your animal. How will they be able to tolerate it?

- Will the benefits outweigh you and your animal going through the process?

Regardless of what path you choose, here are some supportive, natural techniques to use.

Healing Techniques

Sending Love Technique

Titus, a Labrador and pit bull mix, got a cancerous lump on the outside of his nose. When I checked in with the energy of the lump, I saw a lot of anger and hostility. I asked Linetta, Titus' guardian, if she could start sending love to the lump. This was extremely hard for her. Every fiber in her hated it and wanted it gone from his body.

Everything is energy, including a cancerous lump.

I expressed, the cancer is here, so we bless it, receive its message, and then heal it.

This was so hard for Linetta to do. She was clearly upset and mad at the cancer. (That is a natural and normal human response.) It was a mindful, conscious decision for her to shift to connecting, communicating, and sharing love with the cancer.

With the shift in energy and her relationship with the cancerous lump on Titus' nose, it shrank and continued to shrink, and was gone.

Check in with your pet to see if the cancer has a message, what it needs, and what its purpose is to best support the healing.

White Light of Optimum Healing

I first used this technique years ago with my cat, Jessie, and it worked well. Jessie had lung cancer, and with cats hiding their issues so well, I did not know she had it until her breathing was labored. I took her into the emergency veterinarian, who said she had a tumor in her lungs. She was expected to live two days max. Wow, I was devastated.

So, I got on the phone with my animal communication support, (since I was too close to this situation to get accurate and clear information). Jessie was out of body, so with grounding techniques, she got back in her body and received Reiki healing support. I also received communication support with Jessie to see if it was her time to transition. If it were her time, I would accept it. It turns out it was not Jessie's time; however, Jessie did not want to live feeling the way she was feeling. I committed to Jessie I would do my best to support her getting better; and if she did not improve, I would honor her wishes not to live in discomfort. I gave it a week. She was prescribed prednisone. Jessie ran from me, not wanting the pills, so I tossed them into the garbage bin. I was not having my last few moments with Jessie running from me. Daily I held her, visualized her lungs healthy and full of white light energy, breathing with ease. I also gave her craniosacral and energy healing. She made it past the two-day mark and made it to a week, yet her breathing still was heavy, was withdrawn, and still did not feel well. So, in keeping my promise to Jessie not to have her live with discomfort, I called the veterinarian, and scheduled her euthanasia for the next day.

The healing work Jessie had been receiving accumulated, and her body rebounded. The next day, she had easier breathing and much more energy. She was clearly feeling better, so I promptly canceled the euthanasia appointment. I kept working with Jessie, visualizing her lungs healthy, full of white healing light, and breathing easily. I continued giving her craniosacral and energy healing. She lived four more healthy, quality years.

I have been using the White Light of Optimum Health technique ever since on the thousands of clients I have been blessed to serve.

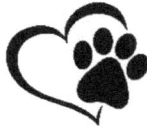

CHAPTER 7

Emergency Support

IN THIS CHAPTER, YOU WILL LEARN techniques to do with your pet in an emergency situation on the way to the veterinarian. These techniques do not replace the need for veterinarian support.

Step-by-Step Instructions

If your pet is in crisis:

1. Call your veterinarian immediately.

2. Get your pet to the veterinarian immediately.

3. Use the following techniques in the veterinarian clinic while waiting for support.

4. If someone else is driving, also use these techniques on the way to the veterinarian.

Support on the Way to Veterinarian

Some techniques and acupressure points for you to do while on the way to the veterinarian (use gentle pressure when holding the acupressure points):

Emergency Resuscitation

From respiratory arrest, sunstroke, or collapse.

- **GV26 Acupressure Point**

  GV26 acupressure point is at the junction where the hairless part of the nose meets the upper lip. Gently touch with steady pressure using your index or middle finger.

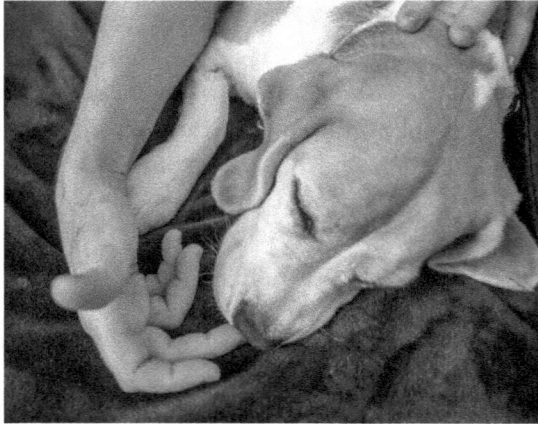

Holding the GV26 Point

Shock Support

- **GV26 Acupressure Point**

  GV26 acupressure point is at the junction where the hairless part of the nose meets the upper lip. Gently touch with steady pressure using your index or middle finger.

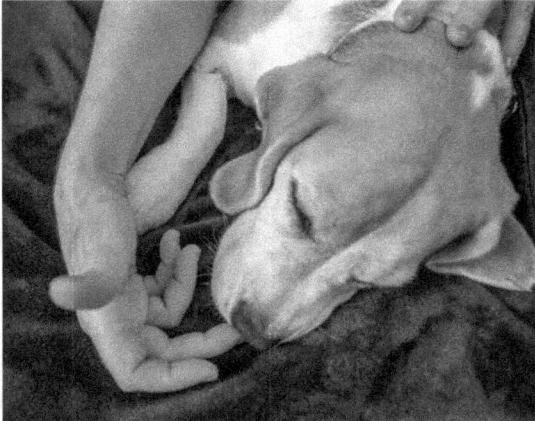

Holding the GV26 Point

- **K1 Acupressure Point**

  The K1 acupressure point is on the hind paws at the base of the pad in the middle of the paw. Gently stimulate this area to activate K1.

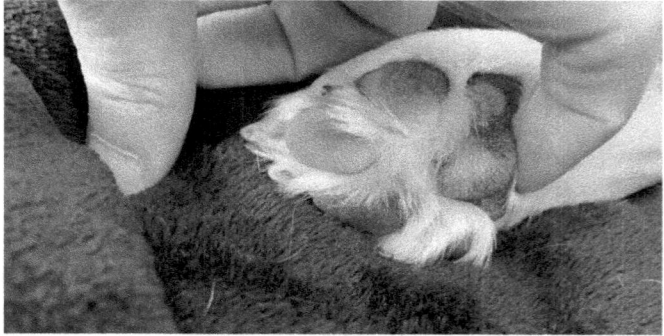

Holding the K1 Point on a Dog

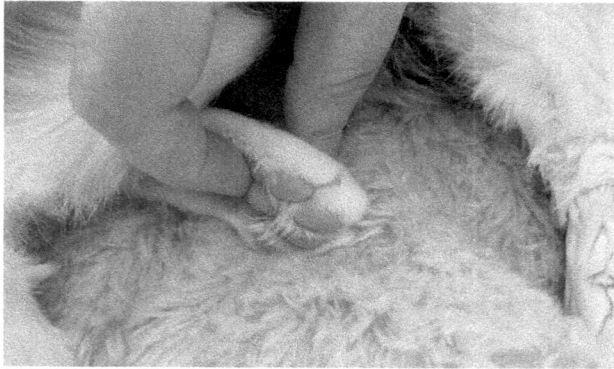

Holding the K1 Point on a Cat

- **HT9 Acupressure Point**

  The HT9 acupressure point is on the front paws at the base of the toenail on the inside of the outer-most toe.

  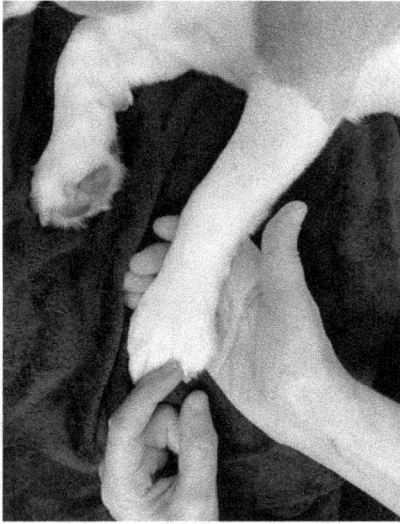

  Holding the HT9 Point

~*Your Essence Experience* ~

*For extra support, the Healing Your Animal **Shock Ease** essence is a natural, effective, easy-to-use way to support your animal in shock. In addition, it will support you to stay grounded as you support your animal in shock. Simply spray the essence three times in the surrounding air to receive grounding support.*

~*Your Essence Experience* ~

*For extra support, the Healing Your Animal **Iceland Spar** essence is a natural, effective, easy-to-use way to get and stay in the present moment. This will support your animal and you as you are in the throes of the emergency. Simply spray the essence three times in the surrounding air to receive balancing support.*

Seizure Support

- **GV20 Acupressure Point**

GV20 acupressure point is recommended to use when your pet is having a seizure, assuming it is safe for you to touch your pet. GV20 is located on the top of the head in the center, between the ears on the front of the bony protuberance. Use light pressure rubbing back and forth with your index or middle finger.

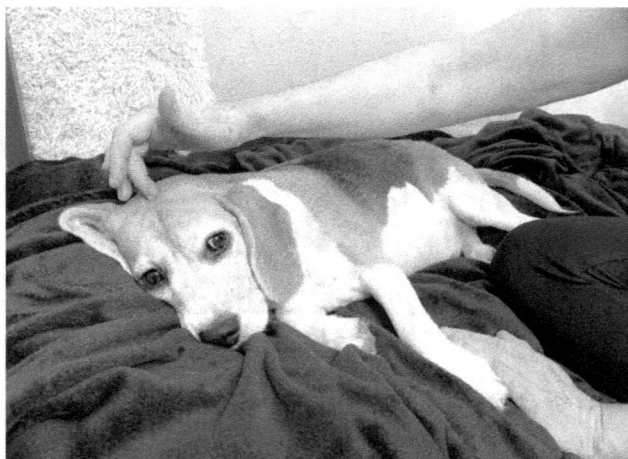

Holding the GV20 Point

- **GB20 Acupressure Point**

GB20 acupressure point is another point to use for seizures. It is located in the nape of the neck, at the base of the skull, immediately behind the back of the ears; find the shallow spot in the arches of the skull.

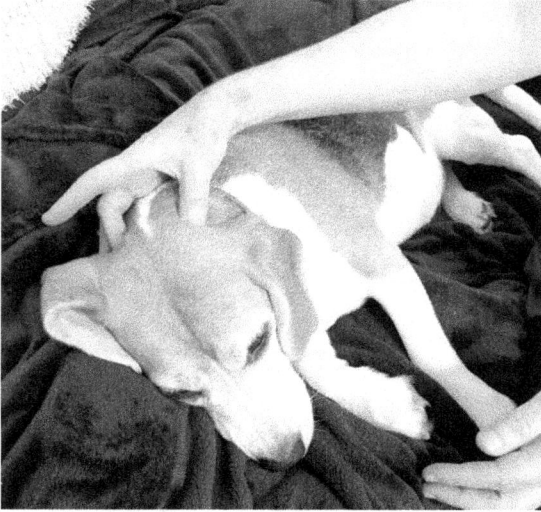

Holding the GB20 Point

☙ *Your Essence Experience* ☙

*For extra support, the Healing Your Animal **Energy Balance** essence is a natural, effective, easy-to-use way to support balancing your animal's energy body. It helps rebalance your animal's energy after having a seizure. Simply spray the essence three times in the air around your animal to receive balancing support.*

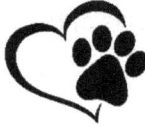

CHAPTER 8

Pain Management and Aging Animals

How to Tell if Your Cat or Your Dog Is in Pain

- Does not jump up on things they used to (couch, bed)
- Hesitates before jumping
- Limping
- Walking slower than normal
- Cannot go for as long of walks as normal
- Not interested in playing or not playing as enthusiastically
- Avoids stairs or jumping in car
- Gives a screech when you touch a certain spot
- Hard to get up from lying position
- Stiff legged
- Anxious, restless

- Sleeping a lot
- Stops on walks and will not go further
- No interest in going for a walk when it is normally fun
- Reactive to certain parts of the body being touched
- Grouchy, grumpy, nippy, may even bite
- Letting out a squeal when touched in specific areas

Example: Not Interested in Going for Normal Fun Walk

I received a call when Sasha, a golden retriever, would not get up for her normal walk. She just stayed on the floor, eyes dull.

It happened that her guardian was out of the country, and the guardian's parents, from England, were pet sitting. Can you imagine being in a foreign country, pet sitting a dog who is normally jumping around to go for a walk who will not get up to go, and being left not knowing what to do or who to call?

Luckily, my information was available to them, and I was able to go check on Sasha. It turned out that Sasha had tight muscles in her back that had gone into spasm and tightened. It was extra uncomfortable for her to move.

After her massage, when her muscles relaxed, she was up bouncing, and perky again, ready for more walks. The sighs of relief all around were huge!

Example: Limping

I was contacted by Lucy's guardian to support Lucy, a senior cat, to feel better and move with ease. Lucy was limping, as she was in discomfort. Lucy was responsive to massage. She had discomfort in her right hip that was causing her to limp. After her massage, she walked straighter and with more vitality.

Managing Pain

When your pet has a soft tissue injury that is fresh and less than 48 hours (two days) old, I recommend that you use the passive touch technique (and Reiki if you are Reiki attuned). The muscles and tissues are in trauma and need to settle before doing any type of massage techniques.

When your pet's injury is over two days old, then you can start using the wellness protocol again and doing the massage techniques for your pet.

Passive Touch

Passive touch increases circulation into the tissue to help cleanse and heal.

Lightly place your whole hand on or just above the injured area of your animal. This light touch that is stationary is called the passive touch massage stroke. It is the only massage stroke that is safe to do on an acute area.

You will have one hand on top of the injured area and one hand on the other side of the injured area, sandwiching the injured area lightly between your hands. This is an extra gentle placement of your hands, as the area may be intensely sensitive to your animal. If you are unable to get two hands around the area, gently place one hand on or slightly above the injured area for healing and comfort.

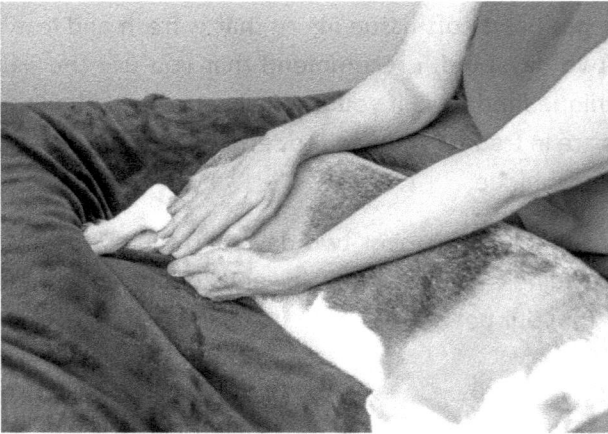
Passive Touch

Massage

Sometimes your pet's behavior is not a clear indication that it is pain related.

Here is a story where massage changed a dog's life. I was volunteering at the Seattle Humane Society, helping animals be adopted that might not have otherwise. They wanted me to work with a nippy dog to see if massage would help calm him so he could be adopted.

He was constantly nipping with fighting, anxious, wiggly, behavior when I was around him and trying to touch him. I was able to work with him despite his unsettled behavior. What I discovered was he had an overly tight muscle on the back of his neck.

As soon as his neck muscle released, he paused, and did a whole-body shake. He immediately quit nipping, pacing, and displaying anxious behavior. He was so calm and relaxed. He was free of his pain. Now he could be adopted.

Shannon first started bringing Scooby, one of her beagle dogs, to see me when Scooby had a neck injury. He had seen his veterinarian, and she had recommended healing sessions with me. His body was radiating heat all through his neck from the muscles being inflamed. He was in a lot of discomfort and was sensitive to being touched on the neck. Shortly after the healing session began, he started settling, as he was getting relief. By the end of his session, he was totally settled.

The healing sessions kept decreasing pain and increasing healing for his neck. Scooby would lie more and more still for his massages. He recovered from his neck injury and received wellness massages throughout the rest of his life.

See Chapter 4 for wellness techniques, including passive touch and massage.

Acupressure

Here are some techniques you can use to relieve pain in your pets:

- **LI4 Acupressure Point**

  Acupressure point LI4 is located inside the first toe, in the web between the dewclaw or where the dewclaw would be. LI4 balances the gastrointestinal system.

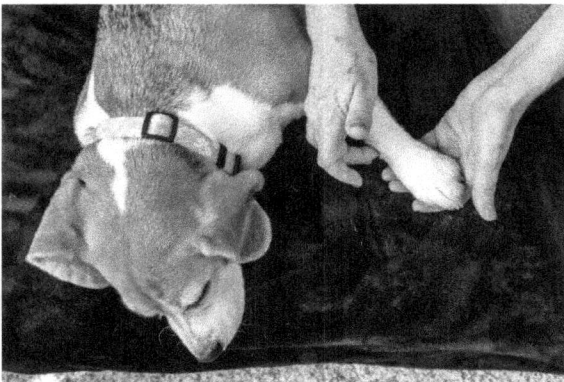

Holding the LI4 Point

- **B60 Acupressure Point**

  Acupressure point B60 is called the aspirin point. It helps with pain relief. Its location is in the depression just above the ankle joint, on the outside of the back leg, between the ankle bone and the Achilles tendon.

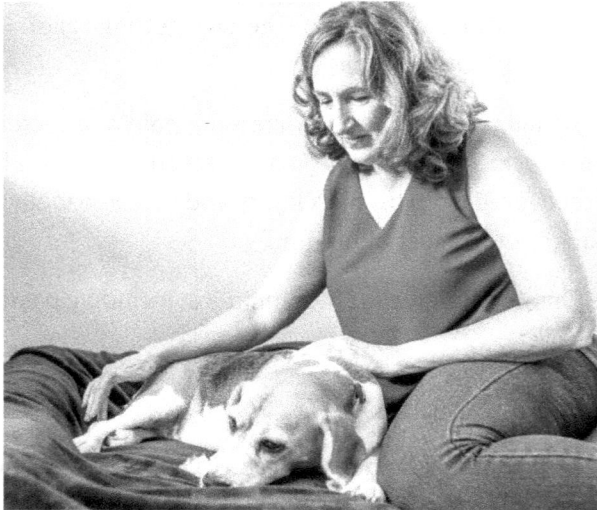

Holding the B60 Point

- **B40 Acupressure Point**

  Acupressure point B40 helps relieve tension in the hind end. Its location is on the back-hind leg, in the very center, right behind the knee. (Acupressure point B40 also labeled B54 in some acupressure charts.)

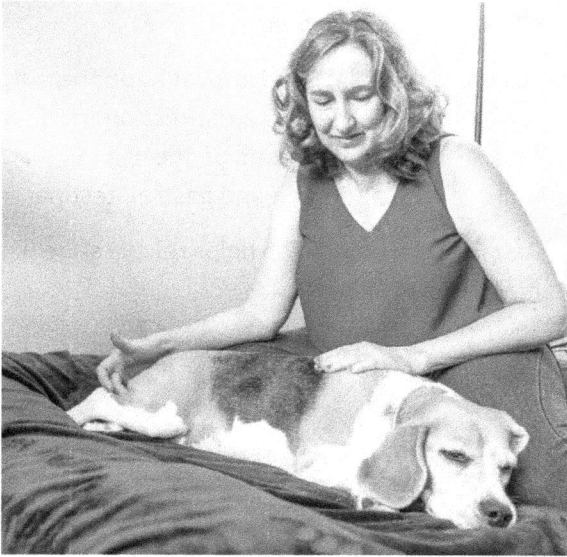

Holding the B40 Point

- **LI10 Acupressure Point**

Acupressure point LI10 supports the front end. The easiest way to find LI10 is to locate LI11 first, then go from there. Lift the front foot, flex the elbow, and you will find a crease forms on the inside of the elbow. Feel for the depression at the end of the crease, now move down the front leg three cun to settle into a point along the bone.

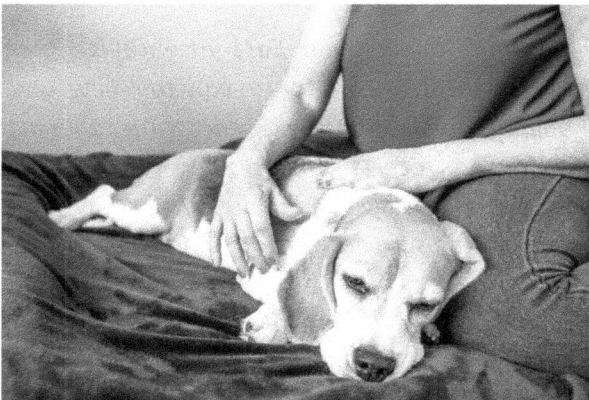

Holding the LI10 Point

- **ST36 Acupressure Point**

  Acupressure point ST36 is located on the outside hind leg, just below the knee, in a depression in the middle of the muscle toward the front of the leg. ST36 is the Master Point for the abdomen and gastrointestinal tract.

  Acupressure point ST36 helps relieve stifle (knee) pain and hind limb weakness.

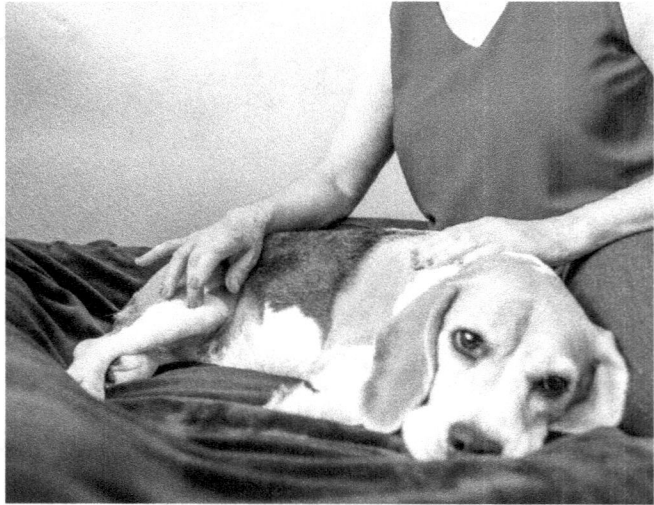

Holding the ST36 Point

ॐ *Your Essence Experience* ॐ

*Healing Your Animal **Pain Ease** essence is a natural, simple, effective, unscented, easy-to-use way to relieve and heal pain for your animal. Simply spray the essence three times in the air around your animal to receive pain-relieving support and benefit from healing support. To give additional relief, spray some in your hand and rub it on the sore area of your animal's body.*

ॐ *Your Essence Experience* ॐ

*Healing Your Animal **Muscle Ease** essence is a natural, simple, effective, unscented, easy-to-use way to relieve and heal muscle* *pain and discomfort for your animal. Simply spray the essence three times in the air around your animal to relieve muscle pain and benefit from healing support. To give additional relief, spray some in your hand and rub it on the sore area of your animal's body.*

*Note: **Pain Ease** and **Muscle Ease** essences are commonly used together for a well-rounded natural pain relief support.*

Aging/Senior Animals

Just like people, animals have more aches and pains as they age. In addition to the wellness healing protocol and the pain management techniques above, here are some techniques to support your senior animal to age gracefully, minimizing pain and increasing quality of life.

Ears

The whole body is supported when you massage your pet's ears.

There are times when an animal client will not let me touch an area on their body that is in pain and discomfort. I have indirect methods of addressing the area of discomfort for them to get relief, and then they will let me touch it. One of these methods is gently massaging the animal's ears. This gives support to the whole body, including the area of discomfort. The extra benefit of massaging the ears for your aging animal is that it stimulates vitality to all areas of your pet's body.

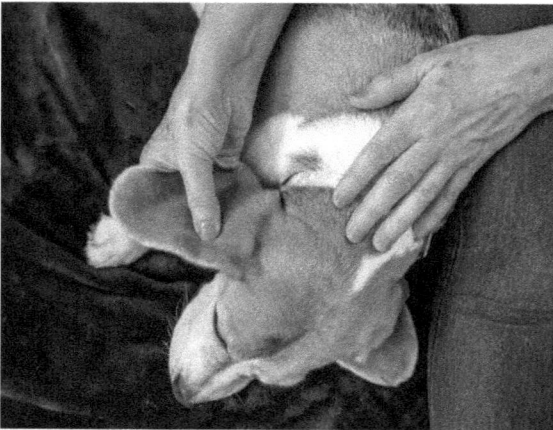
Massaging Ear

Pascal, a Pyrenean Mastiff, was a large, six-month-old puppy who was growing fast. This caused tension and discomfort in his mid-back. He would not let me touch the area to relax the muscles and relieve his discomfort. So, I massaged his ears. Massaging the part of his ear relating to his spine helped give relief to his mid-back. I was then able to palpate and massage the muscles in his mid-back to give him the full relief he needed.

- **SP6 Acupressure Point**

  Acupressure point SP6 is located on the inside of the lower back leg, three cun above the tip of the ankle bone, on the back of the shin bone. SP6 is the Master point for the lower abdomen.

  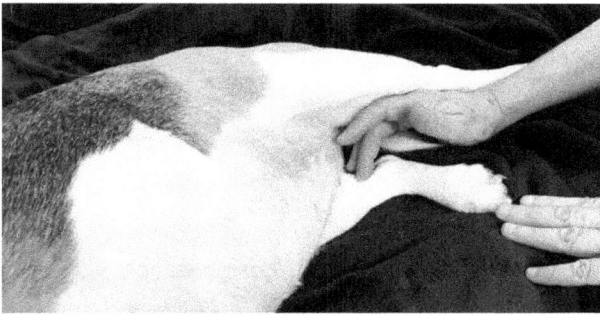

  Holding the SP6 Point

K27 Acupressure Point

Acupressure point K27 is located between the sternum (breastbone) and the first rib, two finger-widths off the ventral (front) midline (center) on each side of the upper chest. It acts as a reset button for your pet's body.

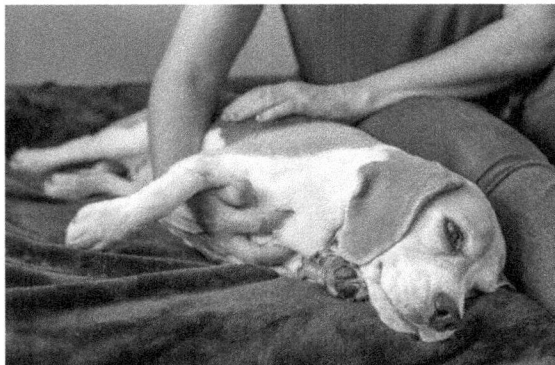

Holding the K27 Point

When Scooby, the beagle, was 14 years old, he was lethargic and sleeping a lot. His energy was depleted. Using the acupressure point K27, he really responded. It helped support his body with more energy and vigor as it was balancing the organs in his body.

Sophie, a five-year-old miniature poodle, would come for healing sessions after her chemotherapy. She would whimper if I supported her with K27 at the beginning of her session. It was too strong for her system. At the end of her healing session, I would support her with K27 to give good balancing to her system. Her body was strong enough to process this acupressure point at the end of her healing session. The nice benefit of acupressure is that it keeps working through the animal's body for 48 hours as it cycles through the 24-hour body clock twice to complete the healing.

∾ *Your Essence Experience* ∾

*Healing Your Animal **Arthritis Ease** essence is a natural, effective, unscented, easy-to-use way to relieve and heal pain for your animal. Simply spray the essence three times in the air around your animal to receive natural pain-relieving support and benefit from healing support. To give additional relief, spray some in your hand and rub it on the sore area of your animal's body.*

*Note: **Arthritis Ease**, **Pain Ease,** and **Muscle Ease** essences are commonly used together for a well-rounded natural pain relief support.*

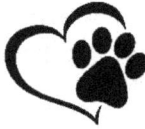

CHAPTER 9

Navigating the End of Your Pet's Life

Having Death Be a Sacred Time

IN MY EXPERIENCE GROWING UP in Western culture, the topic of death was avoided, ignored, and feared. People tended to push their feelings down and act as if it were not happening.

When I grew up, my pets (due to my parents not wanting them in the house) were outside pets. I did sneak them in occasionally and kept being caught. Animals in the wild go off to die, so my pets would just disappear when it was their time. I never knew if they wandered off and were still alive or if they had died. They were just gone. I never had any experience with death until I was an adult with my cat, Tyler.

I thought it was important to educate my daughter, Miranda, on the death and the dying process with animals, as it is a natural part of life. Just as Miranda was turning ten years old, she got a double dose. She lost both of her pets, Sasha, her golden retriever, and

Tasha, her cat, within three weeks of each other. Her father and I gave Miranda the option to be in the room with them or not while they were being put to sleep. She chose to be present for both Sasha's and Tasha's euthanasia. She was extremely brave, being there with them along with both of her parents. Now death is not a mysterious thing for her. She had closure by being there with them.

My belief is that in the death process, the person or animal is transitioning to a new beginning that we do not fully comprehend. It is like when we transition from the womb of our mother into a world we do not know and get to live in the physical world. Death is another transition, a time of rebirth, and new beginnings for the person or animal passing onto their next phase of being. It is a transition and new beginning for those left behind here on Earth.

Death can be honored, and can be a beautiful, sacred process if you choose it to be. You can light candles, have your animal's favorite blanket with them, have their favorite toy by them, share stories with your pet of special times together and how much it has meant to have them in your life. And share your love with them.

My intention is that you gain a deeper understanding to help your animal make the end-of-life journey more peaceful when it is your animal's time to end their time in the physical world.

When Is It Your Animal's Time?

When an animal is diagnosed as sick or dying according to the veterinarian and according to what you see, does not always mean it is the end of life for your animal. If it is not your animal's time to die, they have a chance of rebounding back to health.

I learned this fact at an early age.

I was just 11 years old, when my kitten was diagnosed with distemper and given only a week to live. Rather than accept a tragic diagnosis, I held him in my arms, giving him love. I remember to this day the healing energy kicking in as if time were standing still, with white light surrounding us. My precious kitten rebounded and lived a happy, healthy, and active life for many more years!

I was reminded of it again as an adult with my cat Jessie, who was given two days to live, but lived four more quality years, as you read in Chapter 6.

I have witnessed this rebounding countless times with animals I have had the honor to support with healing over more than 20 years in my private practice.

When it is not a pet's time to transition, it warms my heart to support animals with the gift of extra time and love with their guardians. The extra time I had with my pets was a priceless treasure.

Miracles of Unexpected Recovery

Satchit the Cat

You know it when you have a strong soul connection with your cat. It goes deeper than love. You love all your animals, and when there is one member that has a much stronger heart connection, it goes to the deeper soul level. I call this your "heart" animal (i.e., your heart cat, your heart dog).

Satchit was a 16-year-old cat who was Heather's heart cat. They had a deep soul connection. The veterinarian told Heather that there was nothing more she could do for Satchit, and he was not going to make it. Working with me, Satchit lived another quality year with Heather. This was cherished and priceless to her to have this extra lap time, snuggles, purrs, and companionship with her beloved Satchit.

Mickey the Miracle Kitty

From client Wendy Yellen, Santa Fe, New Mexico

"My cat, Mickey, who has a big heart, was seven years old when she was diagnosed with a liver condition. She was vomiting, horribly yellow from jaundice, and not eating. It came on quickly; I was horrified at seeing her go downhill so far and so quickly. We took her to the veterinarian, who put her in kitty ICU. They really didn't know much they could do, and mostly, they told us, this condition ends in death for cats.

She was on feeding tubes with round-the-clock monitoring, and the veterinarian set the expectation she probably was not going to make it. We visited her every day. I could see Mickey getting sicker and weaker, and this was breaking my heart to think of losing her.

I am no stranger to working with energy healing; I have worked (and trained) with many energy healers around the world. Vicki has enormous skill. So when Vicki communicated with Mickey, and Mickey told Vicki she was going to be coming home again, I did not see how that could happen.

The veterinarian was discussing the possibility of putting her down. Vicki asked that I wait two more days to make that decision, and I agreed. Vicki continued to work with her and during those two days, Mickey started to get visibly stronger. The yellow coloring left, she began eating, and looking like herself again. Very soon after that, Mickey did come home and has been here now for two extra years. She's snuggled in her basket on my desk as I write this, filling my heart with joy. When I took her home, the veterinarian and all the technicians were calling her "the miracle kitty."

Mickey's big heart even touched my husband, who "hates cats." I was absolutely certain he would never touch or pet or talk to a cat, ever. He was adamantly against them. But since then, Mickey won him over. Almost every time he sees her, he picks her up, plays games with her, or feeds her. They have their own special language together. And this would never have happened if Vicki had not been there to support Mickey coming back from death's door, allowing her big heart to literally change the landscape of our home, every day.

Vicki is a loving, passionate, clear, extraordinary presence, and such a gifted and caring healer, for both animals and people who love them."

Tusk the Dog

Tusk, an eight-year-old Bouvier, was diagnosed with bloat and had to have emergency surgery. He was not expected to live through the night. Lynn, Tusk's guardian, called me in, and I went to the doggie ICU to support Tusk. When I walked in, I took one look at Tusk, and my heart immediately sank. He did not look like he was going to make it through the night. Lynn and I supported Tusk with natural healing techniques, including White Light of Optimum Health (see Chapter 6). We stayed until we could feel Tusk stabilize. We knew he was going to live through the night. It was day-by-day progress for him. He kept improving and was able to go home. He lived two and a half more quality years. He even returned to competition for agility titles.

Rebounding is Not Always the Divine Plan

Healing does not always mean getting better. Sometimes the best course of healing for your animal is transitioning to Spirit. In this situation, you can find peace with healing sessions to support your animal in being calmer and reducing suffering, pain, and discomfort.

Asking What Your Animal Wants Is Key

I learned early in my career from a horse named Seven to ask the animal their desire. With Seven, I was putting a lot of energy into getting him better. He would respond during his session and then continue declining. It finally dawned on me to ask Seven what he wanted. Not what his guardian wanted, or I wanted. I supported him with the healing energy to use as he desired. This shift enabled Seven to relax and receive the healing energy fully, and the energy support relieved his pain and discomfort. We were not at odds with our intentions anymore. He received the pain-relieving benefits with ease until he transitioned.

Cerne's Story—A Lesson in Death as Sacred

Early on in my animal healing career, I was asked to support Cerne, an Irish wolfhound, who had been a regular client, with his euthanasia session. At this point, I had never seen an animal die (or a person). I was not quite sure how I would respond; yet something inside of me said I could help, knowing this would change my life and relationships with animals.

When I arrived, Cerne was outside on the lawn, lying and panting with his guardian beside him. I started supporting him with natural pain-relieving techniques, and he calmed down. It was working. His breathing was not as labored. He was getting relief. During this time, his guardian was getting closure with him. The veterinarian arrived. We acknowledged our love for him, and the veterinarian gave Cerne his shots. I felt him peacefully having his last heartbeat and taking his last breath.

It was a beautiful transition, a sacred, blessed event. We were honoring his life. This changed how I viewed death. From feeling scared, out-of-control, and nervous to surrendering, accepting, and blessing the experience.

Thanks to Cerne's teaching, when it came time for my dad to transition, I was able to sit with him, holding love and blessing him and his life. I was able to be there for my dad calmly as he took his last breath, just as I was for Cerne. For this, I am forever grateful.

Cerne's gift was the gift that just kept giving.

I have been able to support many more animals through their passing, and helping their beloved guardians accept and have more peace and connection during their animal's transition.

One client I helped was Sheri Mortko, in Olathe, Kansas, with her first dog, Niko, a whippet, transition as a special, sacred event. After this, Sheri supported multiple family members pass with a beautiful process. And Sheri now volunteers with hospice patients.

What a gift Cerne gave me that has had a ripple effect.

Special Connection Time

When you are connecting with your animal to spend loving, heartfelt, quality time with them, your animal feels this. I invite you to turn off your phone, computer, television, and any other distractions and spend time with your animal.

When they are nearing the end, this is quality time for both of you.

Listed below is a powerful exercise I have used with my own animals and teach to my clients, especially when their animal has received a serious diagnosis, or their animal is nearing the end of life.

Exercise: The Power of Sharing Joy with Your Animals

This exercise is powerful when your animals are healthy, and immensely useful when your animals are preparing to transition. This action helps them understand that you are able to let them transition with ease when it is their time and when it is in their best interest.

The best thing you can do for your animal when you know they do not have much time left is to connect with your animal with love and appreciation. Sit with them and share fun stories and memories of being together.

When I was supporting Sasha, my golden retriever, during hospice, it made a big difference. On the days I used this technique with her, she was thriving, going for walks, and getting the most out of each day. The days I did not use it, Sasha was not interested in walks.

This exercise may be counterintuitive to what you are feeling. It is not easy. As humans, we are sad to be losing our great companions. Most of what we focus on is our grief and sadness. Animals understand that their job is to help us, so they may be confused by our sadness and sometimes think they have done something wrong. They even hold on for us until we have come to terms with their time to go, even though they are in pain or wasting away. That is how much they love us.

Animals are not afraid of death. They inherently accept that it just is when it is their time to go. This is another reason our sadness confuses them.

Please hear me. I am not saying do not feel sad. You are going to feel grief. You are human.

What I am saying is to embrace their living now while they are here. Bring the joy of them into each day, allowing them to feel your love over your awareness of the fact they will be leaving soon.

As I was doing this exercise some days with Sasha, I had tears coming down my face, and I was hugging her, all the while telling her how much joy she brought me. I tried to keep that focus on one level, while I was in deep pain on another. She could still feel my love.

This exercise will provide more quality-bonding togetherness with you and your special, wonderful furry friend.

I invite you to use this with your cats and your dogs. And let me know what happens.

(I share this exercise on an episode of my Animal Messages podcast: The Power of Sharing Joy When Your Pet Is Passing.)

Peace, Comfort, and Great Bonding

One of the greatest benefits is having support in place before your animal transitions. Here is a guideline I use to help my clients when their animal is in the dying process:

The dying process of your precious pet is an emotional time for you as a guardian. It may be hard for you to communicate clearly with your animal at this time. I am sharing my process and recommend that you get support from a professional animal communicator/healer or myself for greater peace.

Support I put in place before the animal transitions:

- Understand the animal's wishes.

- Help the guardian make a plan.

- Manage the animal's pain and add comfort.

- Build a bridge of light. This healing technique helps your animal cross over to the other side with ease.

- Share communication between the guardian and animal, so everything is clear.

- Establish a sign from the animal how they will let their guardian know it is them connecting from the Spirit world.

This gives guardians peace and comfort and is a great bonding experience before their animal passes.

Create your pet's passing to be a blessed, sacred event. You can have candles, your pet's favorite blanket, favorite toy, soft music, and share lots of love. You are celebrating them for being in your life. Celebrating how much they blessed you with their love and presence, and how much you loved them. Those memories live on forever.

Things to Consider with Decision Time

Whether it is your first experience with an animal transitioning, it is never easy, and it is never the same.

Here are common questions that arise:

- Am I doing all I can do to help my animal?
- Will my pet pass on his/her own?
- Do I need to make the decision to euthanize my pet?
- When is the time to make that decision?
- Am I killing my pet before his/her time?
- What if it is too soon? Will my animal forgive me?
- What if it is not what my animal wants?
- Is my pet suffering?
- What am I going to do without him/her?
- I cannot bear to lose him/her yet. Is my pet hanging on for me?

Every animal is unique, and so is their transitioning process. There is no one definite model to follow, which makes the decision process feel like you are on an emotional roller coaster.

One day your animal may be perky, the next day extra low energy and withdrawn, and then the next day perky again. It is a day-by-day, moment-to-moment experience. It can be exhausting, unsettling, and a time of uncertainty. One way for you to know it is time is you will see it in your animal's eyes. They will be dull, listless, and almost vacant looking.

You desire to live without regret and have peace of mind, knowing you did all you could to give your pet the best care and best life, and that you made the best decision for with euthanasia at the right time.

I know I wanted my cat, Tyler, to die on his own. He was my first pet that I had to make the decision to euthanize. He was hanging on for me. Even though I was telling him he had permission to pass (and I truly was hoping he would, so I did not have to make the decision), he did not. He was wasting away. He had gotten down to four pounds, and he was too weak to jump or walk very far, could barely lift his paw up to connect, and that is when I knew I had to take the matter into my own hands for him.

I was at the veterinarian, crying, talking, and asking all the questions you have asked if you have gone through this process. I was so scared I was putting him down too early. I wondered if a miracle would happen and he would rebound and have more life to live.

Once the veterinarian talked with me about the truth of what was happening in Tyler's gut and the dire implications of it, I made the decision to euthanize Tyler right then. I got the biggest gift of all. When Tyler's spirit left his body, he circled me, wrapping himself around me twice as a thank you and nurturing gesture. Then he paused for a moment, flying above me, showing me he was happy and free, and then went off to where spirits go when they transition. His affection showed me his thanks for helping him be free from his physical body and the pain and discomfort he was in. I knew it was the right thing to do for him. I was and still am immensely grateful for his teaching in that moment.

I later realized why he was hanging on. I had three cats, two females and one male, Tyler. I had recently divorced and was calling him the "man of the house." I was single, not seeing anyone, and he took his role seriously. He did not want to leave me with no "man of the house."

If you think your animals do not care what you call them or say to them, think again. They take your words to heart and their roles seriously.

Your Pets as Teachers

Sheri did not grow up around dogs. When Niko, a whippet, came into her life, she was learning from him about dogs.

When she was selecting her puppy, Niko connected with her, watched her with the other puppies, and was happy when Sheri noticed him. He was right there waiting for Sheri to realize that he was her puppy, and she was his person.

Since Niko was Sheri's first dog, it was her first time to go through death with a pet when it was his time.

When Niko was 10 years old, he was diagnosed with cancer. It was too far along for treatment. Sheri had more time with Niko through the death process, supporting him with love, Western medicine, and natural healing energy sessions.

She was grateful that Niko and I had a healing relationship before he got sick. Niko knew me and could trust me as I helped him navigate this journey. Sheri was interested in making sure Niko was not afraid and was not in pain.

In our sessions, we would check in on issues Niko was experiencing. I taught Sheri the techniques to use with Niko that I am teaching in this book to relieve pain, relieve nausea, relieve digestive discomfort, and increase comfort.

Niko would go from some enjoyment to getting tired easily.

Sheri was aware of the dimming of his energy and the light in his eyes, energy fading and getting brighter, expanding, and contracting.

She commented she would have dismissed it or condemned it without our work together. At the end, it was clear that Niko's energy had faded to the point that she needed not to ask him to stay.

Sheri engaged fully in connection with Niko. She was watching him and helping him die with love. This was truly a heart-to-heart connection for them. She was learning from Niko about the death process.

Sheri had fixed beliefs that she was able to get rid of with Niko. Sheri had a fear that when Niko passed, he would disappear. He did not.

Niko understood and was willing to help Sheri learn how it works by coming back and connecting from the other side. Niko taught Sheri that animals leave physically, but they are not gone.

Still, there are tears of grieving and sadness.

According to Sheri, the worst part of having an animal is when you have to give them back. It is not that a new love fixes the heartbreak at all.

The new love she is talking about is Farrah, another whippet. While Farrah can never replace Niko, Perry, or Levi, Farrah is a blessing in Sheri's life.

Blessings Between a Pet and Her Person

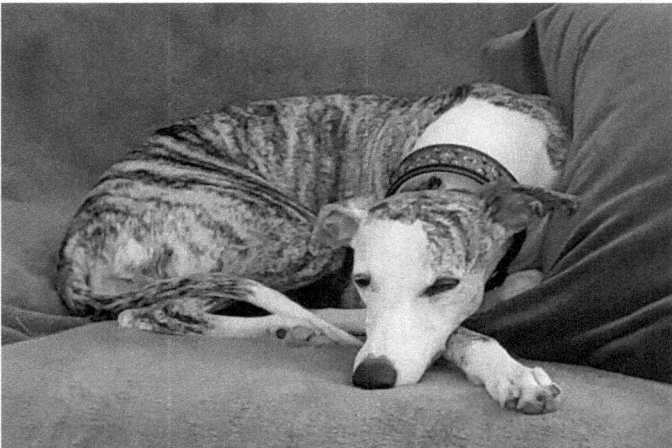

Farrah—photo submitted by Sheri Mortko

Farrah had just turned three and had just had a litter of eight puppies. She was still lactating when she came to Sheri because her breeder fell and broke her ankle when these puppies were just seven and a half weeks old. The breeder and all the puppies went to Kentucky to live with a family who could take care of them all.

Farrah, under normal circumstances, would have been with her puppies for the first twelve to sixteen weeks. Life is not always ideal.

Sheri received her cancer diagnosis about the time the COVID-19 pandemic started. She got a double whammy.

It was Divine alignment that Farrah was there for Sheri to navigate cancer.

Farrah had just turned five at the time of this interview with Sheri.

"Even though Farrah was not in a shelter or in horrible circumstances, I rescued Farrah, and she knows it. At the breeder's home, Farrah was not allowed on the furniture, she was not allowed to cuddle; she was just a piece of furniture. This breeder was done with her. They were friends; they were not family. As soon as Farrah was old enough, she left her breeder, went to a handler, and was in her show life. For Farrah to finally realize that I am her person, and she is not going to be shuttled and shuffled around anymore is a gift.

"I can see how relieved Farrah is to live here with us. And how grateful and how she finally got what she was looking for, and that feels magical.

"She is not super high energy or high drive. She is very mellow and laid back. And that is what I needed to have during my cancer surgery and recovery time."

It was Divine alignment that Sheri was there to give Farrah a loving home.

Remember to Share Love With Your Healthy Pet

Sometimes you have another healthy pet still with you as one is getting sick, declining, and transitioning.

During this process, it is important to give the healthy pet positive attention as you are supporting your sick pet that is taking much of your attention.

Shannon had two beagles, Scooby and Gracie, who were regular clients. They initially started seeing me when Scooby had a neck injury. When I was giving Scooby a massage, Gracie was in the room lying near, soaking up the healing energy, and sighing when Scooby had a release, a healing shift in processing his session. Gracie was helping and receiving at the same time, even though the session's focus was on Scooby. This led to Gracie receiving her own session. When Scooby got cancer, Gracie was still getting some attention, while Scooby received most of the focus. This helped Gracie understand the process and feel a part of the process.

In the event of death, it is important to give your pet still living positive attention as you are grieving the loss.

Your living pet is grieving too and is concerned about you and trying to help you process your grief. This energy can get stuck in them. It would be helpful for you to have a healing session to clear your grief from your pet's body to maintain wellness. An animal communication session supports your living pet to understand and process your other pet's death.

Gracie had a session after Scooby's passing, to help Gracie clear her grief and understand her guardian's grief.

Shannon and Scooby had a big heart and soul connection, and Shannon's grief ran deep. A month after Scooby's passing, I was back seeing Gracie. With Gracie receiving support, she understood her guardian's grieving, and it relieved any worry or concern from Shannon about Gracie while she took care of herself.

❧ *Your Essence Experience* ❧

*For extra support, the Healing Your Animal **Transition** essence is a natural, effective, easy-to-use way to support your pet and you while navigating the dying process with your animal. Simply spray the essence three times in the surrounding air to receive healing support.*

End-of-Life Support for You and Your Animal

There is a natural grieving process that you go through with the loss of your pet. Grieving is different for every individual. It is a time to be kind, loving, and nurturing to yourself.

I have other techniques I use to help you and your pet through the dying process that are beyond the scope of this book. I teach these to private clients and in classes. If this is something you desire to learn, please get in touch with me at HealingYourAnimal.com.

❧ *Your Essence Experience* ❧

*For extra support, the Healing Your Animal **Pain Ease** essence is a natural, effective, easy-to-use way to relieve physical and emotional pain. It is supportive during the journey of your pet dying and after your pet has transitioned. It provides a calming, nurturing balm to your hurting heart. Simply spray the essence three times in the surrounding air to receive healing support.*

Bereavement Support

Another resource to reach out to is AHelp Project, (AHelpProject.org). AHELP is the Animal Hospice, End-of-Life, and Palliative Care Project.

Michelle Nikols is the Founder of AHelp Project, and her mission is to expand animal hospice and teach more people about it.

Michelle is not a licensed mental health therapist; she is a grief and bereavement counselor, so she connects people with resources for intensive therapy and ongoing therapy to get through the grief of losing a pet.

When interviewing Michelle, I asked her, "What is the biggest thing you can offer someone whose pet is on death's door?" Michelle's reply was:

"Spend quality time with your pet, it is the time to get down on the floor, get in a chair with them on your lap, get in a space where it is just you and your pet, and make sure you impart love on him/her. It is about quality of life until the end of life.

Sudden death or when an animal goes missing is the worst grief to process."

Michelle is a grief and bereavement counselor; she can help you process your grief. If you need more intensive support, she can get you resources for your needs.

None of us knows when our pet's time is, so it is important to make the best of each moment.

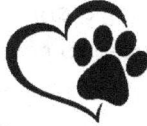

CHAPTER 10

Heart to Heart Daily Connection, Joy, and Gratitude with Your Animal

SHARING YOUR LIFE WITH A PET is one of the most rewarding parts of life. You have a special bond, unconditional love, and unique personalities.

This chapter is how to get the most of your connection with your pet every day, so when it is their time to cross over, you have cherished, enjoyed, and made the most of your time together.

Connecting Moments With Your Pet

Sometimes your animal connects with you in a way you may not like. For instance, Spirit, my kitty, was rejected by his mom at one day old. He has a strong need to lick, nibble, and connect. And he is also a drooler. This is my first experience with a drooling kitty.

Miranda, my daughter, and I have termed this behavior as his "love mode." When he gets into it, he is purring, he is focused, he is determined to connect, lick my face, nibble on my earlobe (nibble is a nice term for sometimes chomping on it), and rubbing his face against mine, getting drool all over my face while kneading his paws on my chest. I used to get really irritated with him, as I did not like this. I would push him away, and he would jump right back. He was determined to get his needs met. I was unable to find a toy or something to deflect this behavior. So, I decided to turn it into calling it "love mode," open my heart, and connect with him, as he needs to have this connection to get a basic need filled. Now he ends up purring and sitting with me, connecting heart to heart, reducing the nibbling on my earlobe and drooling on my face. This decision to listen to his needs turned an irritating connection with Spirit into a precious, loving connection that has shifted our quality of bonding.

Sapphire and I have developed our connection too. She is not a traditional lap kitty. When I am doing self-Reiki or meditating, Sapphire is attracted to the energy and immediately jumps in my lap, rubs up against me, and lies down. Meditating is traditionally practiced in a room with no distractions. I have found during this connection with Sapphire that I can meditate and have our connection without it being a distraction. And it warms my heart to have this bonding activity.

Playful and Present

Your pet is always in the present moment.

An article in Psychology Today[1] says we are present about 50% of the time in life. Wow, that is a lot of time spent in the past or future.

---

[1] Psychology Today, "New Study Shows Humans Are on Autopilot Nearly Half the Time," by David Rock, posted November 14, 2010

The past is where the mind usually remembers negative emotions. The future has not happened yet, so there is worry, fear, and anxiety about it.

Both modern research and ancient wisdom say being present is the only place to be truly happy.

Did you know when you are playing, you are 100% present?

It is time for more play!

Health Benefits of Play

According to HelpGuide.org, the benefits of play for adults include the following[2]:

1. Play relieves stress, decreases inflammation, and increases vascular health. Play releases endorphins, the body's natural feel-good chemical. Another benefit is that play temporarily relieves pain.

2. Play improves brain function. Puzzle games, chess, and games that stimulate your thinking prevent memory problems. The social interaction wards off stress and depression.

3. Play stimulates the mind and boosts creativity. You learn a new task better when it is fun, and you are relaxed in a playful mood.

4. Play improves relationships and your connection to others. Sharing laughter and fun can foster empathy, compassion, trust, and intimacy with others. It does not have to be an activity; it can be a state of mind. A playful

---

[2] HelpGuide.org, "The Benefits of Play for Adults," by Lawrence Robinson, Melinda Smith, M.A., Jeanne Segal, Ph.D., and Jennifer Shubin. Last updated: October 2020.

nature helps you loosen up in stressful situations, break the ice with strangers, and make new friends.

5. Play keeps you young and energetic. It boosts energy and vitality, and even improves your resistance to disease, helping you function at your best.

6. Play can heal emotional wounds. Play means you are having fun and your pet is having fun.

What do you do for play?

How often?

Is there something you can do daily to spark more joy and play in your day-to-day life?

Exercise: Being Present

- Put your cell phone away.
- Focus on your pet.
- Connect through play with your pet.
- Notice your pet's reaction when you play and are having fun.

Exercise: Heart Connecting

Your animals are pure unconditional love. The heart center is where your animals are always open and connecting, and patiently waiting for you to connect with them at this deep level.

A good daily practice for having heart-to-heart connection is:

- Pause.

- Get present by breathing three deep breaths in and out.

- Put your hand on your heart (center of your chest) to connect in, shift from your head to your heart, and open your heart center.

- Connect with your pet from this space, and talk, hug, rub, or play.

Playtime With Your Pet

Each animal is unique and has his/her preferences for what thrills them with play. As a loving pet guardian, you get to discover what your pet likes and dislikes, and provide stimulation for what they like.

Examples of Indoor Games

Bubbles: See if your pet likes chasing bubbles. I have had both cats and dogs who liked playing with bubbles floating through the air as I created them. Be sure the bubbles you use are safe for pets.

Toys: Toys help keep your pet mentally stimulated. Toys come in many shapes and sizes. You get to have the adventure of discovery about what toys your pet is drawn to and really likes.

Treats: You can make a game out of hiding treats and letting your pet find them. Toys filled with treats that come out when the toy is played with provide entertainment for both cats and dogs. There are multiple puzzle games for treats for both cats and dogs. Check them out in your local pet store or online.

For cats: Catnip, crinkle, and wand toys are some examples of cat-specific toys. One of my cats likes things that move on the ground, and one likes to jump for things. They play with some common toys, and I have others that each of them prefers to help keep them engaged.

For dogs:

- **Chase:** Your dog may like a good game of chase with you or just run around with you for a fun, connecting activity.

- **Frisbee:** Some dogs like to play Frisbee. You can see if your dog is up for a game.

- **Fetch:** Some dogs like to play fetch. This can be tossing a ball or stick on dry ground or in the water.

Exercise: Jumping For Joy

Put on your favorite song. Start dancing and jumping for joy, and watch what happens with your animals.

From someone who gets serious when I am focused, I decided to loosen up.

Doing healing sessions is playful energy for me. However, when I am working on the parts of my business and life that are not in a healing session environment, I tend to get excessively serious and focused. In order to loosen up, I put on a song that makes me happy and start dancing with joy.

When I first did this with my golden retriever, Sasha, I looked over, and she got a big sparkle in her eyes, jumped up from where she was lying, and she started dancing around with me. Both of us were full of life and joy. We were having the best time. I could see joy in her, I was feeling joy, and it was something we were doing together. I was having fun, and it was fun seeing the effect on her.

She was having a fantastic time bouncing and engaging and doing this with me. That was so memorable.

As a human, I can get back in my pattern of being too serious, and realize I need to make this a part of my regular life and self-care to lighten up and play more. I am sure I am not the only one, so I am sharing this message from Sasha to experience joy with your pet. It means a lot to them, and the memories are so heart-warming for me.

I did this recently with my cats, Spirit and Sapphire. I set the intention that I was jumping for joy and inviting them to participate. Sapphire was drawn to the joy energy; she came over and lay down and rolled over, so I bent down and rubbed her belly. She loved it. Spirit, seeing this with Sapphire, decided to join in. They were closely engaged and connecting in their cat way.

I invite you to do this and see what your pet does.

❧ Your Essence Experience ❧

*For extra support, the Healing Your Animal **Play** essence is a natural, effective, easy-to-use way to embrace play and enhance childhood wonder. Simply spray the essence three times in the air surrounding to receive playful support.*

❧ Your Essence Experience ❧

*For extra support, the Healing Your Animal **Embrace** essence is a natural, effective, easy-to-use way to embrace your authentic self with protection as you grow spiritually. Simply spray the essence three times in the surrounding air to receive healing support.*

❧ Your Essence Experience ❧

*For extra support, the Healing Your Animal **Reflection** essence is a natural, effective, easy-to-use way to show your highest self to the world and have it be reflected back to you. Simply spray the* *essence three times in the surrounding air to receive healing support.*

For more techniques on how to help you and your precious pets live your best lives, full of health, harmony, and happiness, I invite you to look for my next book: *"Healthy, Free, and Harmonious: Balancing Your and Your Pet's Chakras"*.

It has truly been an honor to be joined with you and your animals in support of having you and your animals be in optimum health, harmony, connection, and peace.

—Vicki Draper, Author, Certified Healer
and Animal Communicator.

Sending you many hugs with lots of love, purrs, and woofs!

Resources

Podcast

Animal Messages—What Your Animal Wants You To Know with Host Vicki Draper: anchor.fm/vicki-draper9

Shelters/Rescue Organizations

Boston Terrier Rescue of Western Washington: btrww.org

Feral Care Sanctuary feralcaresanctuary.org

Meow: meowcatrescue.org

NOAH Center: thenoahcenter.org

Pasado's Safe Haven: pasadosafehaven.org

Purrfect Pals: purrfectpals.org

Seattle Humane Society: seattlehumane.org

Seattle Purebred Dog Rescue: spdrdogs.org/

Education

Healing Your Animal: healingyouranimal.com

Northwest School of Animal Massage: nwsam.com

Tallgrass Animal Acupressure: animalacupressure.com

Grief Support

AHelp Organization: aHelpProject.org

Nutrition

Natural Pet Pantry: naturalpetpantry.com

Whole Cat & Kaboodle: thewhole-cat.com

Quality Essential Oils, Floral Waters & Others

Aromatics international: aromatics.com

Levensboom: levensboom.com

Florihana: florihana.com/us

Boswellness: boswellness.com

Oshandhi: oshandhi.co.uk

NHR Organics: nhrorganicoils.com

Certified Aromatherapists

Before you work with an aromatherapist, ask if they use natural aromatherapy products.

Northwest School of Animal Massage: NWSAM.com

Current therapists: Joan Sorita, Julie Duke, and Erika Ray

National Association of Natural Aromatherapy: Naha.org

Acupressure Charts

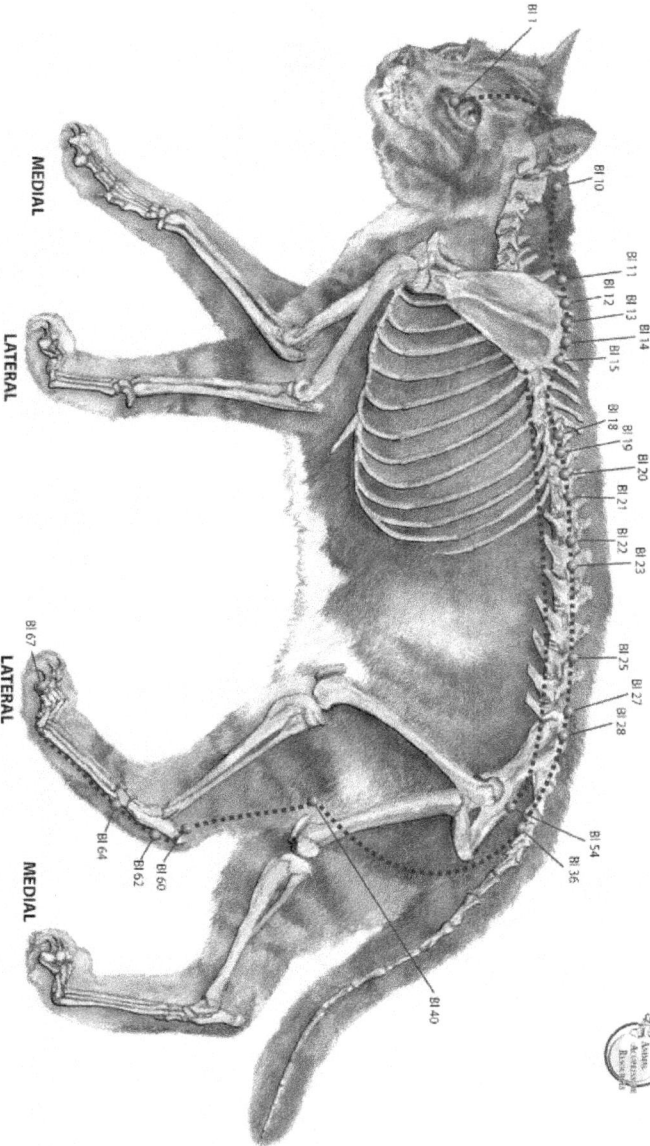

Feline Bladder Meridian Chart ©2020

MEDIAL

LATERAL

LATERAL

MEDIAL

Bl 1
Bl 10
Bl 11
Bl 12
Bl 13
Bl 14
Bl 15
Bl 18
Bl 19
Bl 20
Bl 21
Bl 22
Bl 23
Bl 25
Bl 27
Bl 28
Bl 54
Bl 36
Bl 40
Bl 67
Bl 64
Bl 62
Bl 60

Canine Bladder Meridian Chart ©2020

Vicki Draper

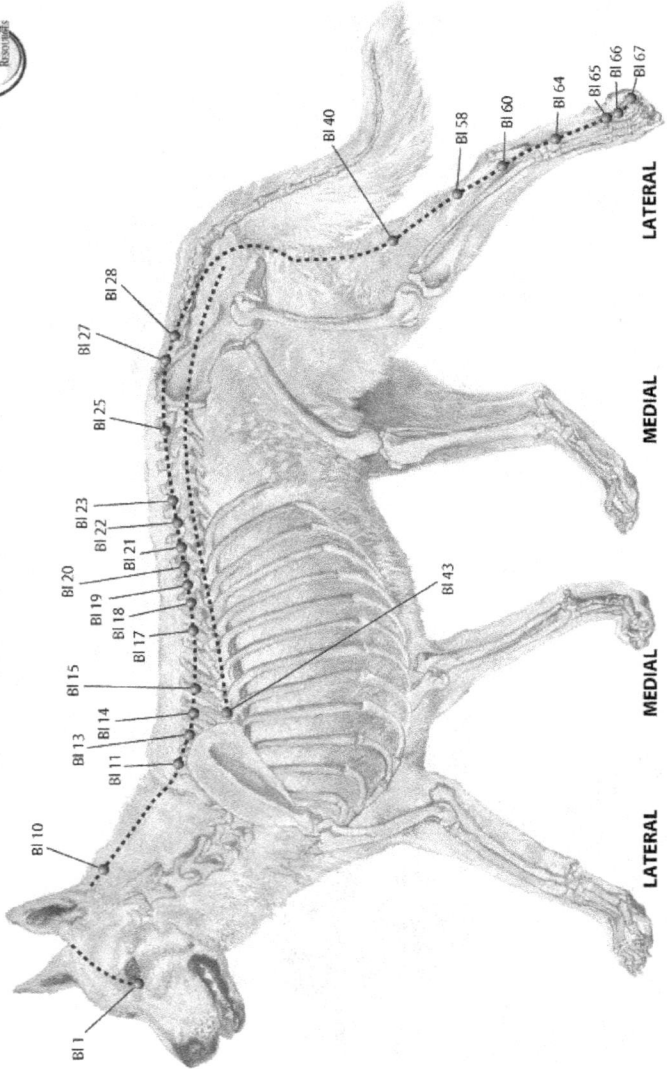

BI 1
BI 10
BI 11
BI 13
BI 14
BI 15
BI 17
BI 18
BI 19
BI 20
BI 21
BI 22
BI 23
BI 25
BI 27
BI 28
BI 40
BI 43
BI 58
BI 60
BI 64
BI 65
BI 66
BI 67

LATERAL
MEDIAL
MEDIAL
LATERAL

Acupressure Charts: Permission was granted by Nancy Zidonis and Amy Snow of Tallgrass Animal Acupressure Resources authors of *ACU-DOG: A Guide to Canine Acupressure, ACU-CAT: A Guide to Feline Acupressure,* and *ACU-HORSE: A Guide to Equine Acupressure.* They founded Tallgrass Animal Acupressure Resources, which offers books, manuals, DVDs, apps, meridian charts and many more acupressure learning tools.

Contact: animalacupressure.com, tallgrass@animalacupressure.com
Note: Vicki Draper is a graduate of the Tallgrass training program and received her certification in equine and small animal acupressure.

Gratitude

Years ago, at a spiritual workshop, I received the intuitive guidance that my purpose here on Earth and my lesson was Love.

This book Heart to Heart has truly been a growth in opening my heart wider, being able to receive more love and express more love. Not only expressing and giving more love in the healing sessions, in my life as well.

I am grateful for all of the animals who have been part of my life, being a guardian for, supporting with healing, having brief encounters, and the joy of seeing them playful and being themselves full of joy.

I am grateful for wildlife support, to the eagle who came for the Grounded While Soaring Essence creation, to the minerals and crystals of the Earth that have come for supporting you and your animals along with me with healing through the essences, through nature's inspiration, through all of my human and animal teachers on this journey, to God for my spark and passion, and to COVID-19's isolation and loss for helping me open my heart more and really connecting to what truly matters.

Thank you Center for Spiritual Living Seattle and prayer practitioner licensing, thank you to all of the practitioner prayer support team, thank you to all of the animals, and thank you to my teachers receiving my licensing and certifications in addition to the spiritual gifts and guidance enabling me to assist millions of people and animals live happy, healthy, and harmonious lives.

I am also grateful to all of the people and animals in my life who have benefitted from using these healing techniques that are now helping you have a deeper heart-to-heart connection and healthier life with your animals.

About the Author

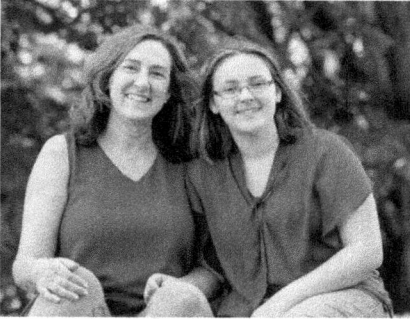

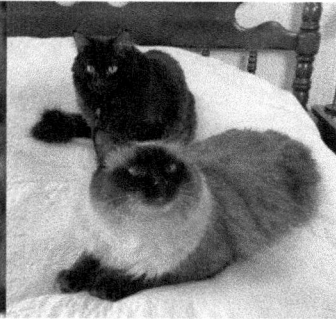

Vicki Draper is a highly regarded modern-day animal healer and author who supports family animals with health, harmony, and ease addressing wellness during every stage of your animal's life. With her skill set, she serves people locally and remotely, nationally and internationally.

She is featured in multiple books and magazines and is the creator of healing products sold around the country and around the world. A natural-born animal communicator, Vicki's qualifications as a healer for both people and animals, include being a licensed massage practitioner, a certified acupressurist and Reiki Master/Teacher, and training in craniosacral therapy.

Vicki deepened her connection with spirituality and was called to become a Science of Mind Prayer Practitioner with the Center for Spiritual Living in Seattle. She is trained and licensed to support others to face life challenges through affirmative prayer, which helps her better serve animals and their human families.

Vicki lives in the Greater Seattle Area with her two cats, Spirit and Sapphire, and Miranda when she is visiting from college. She loves to walk in nature daily, connecting with herons, eagles, and wildlife, bringing nature's wisdom into her life and healing practice.

If you would like further assistance with yourself or your animals, Vicki invites you to schedule a Healing Your Animal Assessment, to discuss your issues and concerns and together determine the best plan of support.

Connect with Vicki at HealingYourAnimal.com

www.ingramcontent.com/pod-product-compliance
Lightning Source LLC
Chambersburg PA
CBHW070913270326
41927CB00011B/2556